Biochemistry

Azhar ul Haque Sario

AF706127

Copyright

Copyright © 2026 by Azhar ul Haque Sario

All rights reserved. No part of this book may be reproduced in any manner whatsoever without written permission except in the case of brief quotations embodied in critical articles and reviews.
First Printing, 2026

Azhar.sario@hotmail.co.uk

ORCID: https://orcid.org/0009-0004-8629-830X
LinkedIn: https://www.linkedin.com/in/azharulhaquesario/

Disclaimer: This book is free from AI use. The cover was designed in Canva.

Copyright Disclaimer: This book is an independently produced educational resource by Azhar ul Haque Sario. It is not affiliated with, endorsed by, or connected to any specific examination board, university, or official curriculum body. Any use of trademarks, brand names, or specific curriculum terms is for descriptive, nominative fair use purposes only, to help readers identify the relevant subject matter.

Contents

BIOCHEMISTRY OF CELL

Part 1: The Importance of Biochemistry in Dentistry

Biochemistry is the bridge between the inanimate world of chemistry and the vibrant world of biology. In dentistry, it is the foundation upon which all diagnosis, prevention, and material science rests.

1.1 The Oral Cavity as a Biochemical Ecosystem

The mouth is often described as a mirror of the body, but biochemically, it is more like a battlefield. It is the only place in the human body where hard mineralized tissues (enamel) are constantly exposed to the external environment, including bacteria, fermentable sugars, and temperature fluctuations.

The Salivary "Liquid Biopsy" For decades, we viewed saliva merely as a digestive aid. In 2026, we recognize saliva as a "diagnostic powerhouse"—a liquid biopsy that rivals blood testing.

Buffering Capacity: Saliva contains the bicarbonate buffer system ($HCO3^-$), which neutralizes acids produced by bacteria. Without this biochemical shield, teeth would dissolve within weeks.

Diagnostic Biomarkers: Modern dentistry uses salivary diagnostics to detect systemic diseases. We can now identify specific RNA markers and exosomes (tiny vesicles) in saliva that indicate early-stage diabetes, oral cancer, and even cardiovascular stress.

Viral Reservoirs: Post-pandemic research has cemented the understanding of salivary glands as reservoirs for viral replication, changing how we approach infection control biochemically.

Clinical Relevance: When you see a patient with "rapidly progressing caries," do not just drill and fill. Ask yourself: Is their biochemical buffering capacity compromised? Are their salivary proteins (like statherin) failing to maintain calcium supersaturation?

1.2 Hard Tissue Biochemistry: The Tug-of-War

Enamel is the hardest substance in the human body, composed of 96% inorganic mineral. This mineral is Hydroxyapatite ($Ca_{10}(PO_4)_6(OH)_2$). However, this crystal is not static. It is in a constant state of flux.

The Critical pH Concept The chemical stability of enamel is governed by pH.

Demineralization: When oral bacteria (like S. mutans) metabolize sugar via glycolysis, they excrete lactic acid. When the local pH drops below 5.5 (the critical pH), the phosphate ions in the saliva can no longer keep the enamel crystal stable. The equation shifts to the right, and the tooth begins to dissolve.

$$Ca_{10}(PO_4)_6(OH)_2 + 8H^+ \rightarrow 10Ca^{2+} + 6HPO_4^{2-} + 2H_2O$$

Remineralization: This is the natural repair process. If the pH rises back to neutral, calcium and phosphate ions from saliva precipitate back into the tooth surface, reforming the crystal lattice.

Fluoride: The Ionic Imposter Fluoride is the ultimate biochemical "hack." When fluoride ions (F^-) are present in the mouth, they substitute for the hydroxyl group (OH^-) in the hydroxyapatite crystal.

This creates Fluorapatite ($Ca_{10}(PO_4)_6F_2$).

Why is this important? Fluorapatite is chemically more stable and less soluble than natural enamel. Its critical pH is lower (around 4.5), meaning the bacteria have to work much harder and produce much more acid to dissolve this "upgraded" enamel.

1.3 The Biochemistry of Caries and Periodontal Disease

Dental Caries (Tooth Decay) Caries is not a hole in the tooth; it is a metabolic disease. It is caused by a dysbiosis—an imbalance in the biofilm (plaque).

Glycolysis: Cariogenic bacteria ingest sucrose and use the enzyme Invertase to split it. They then run the glucose through the glycolytic pathway to generate ATP (energy) and lactic acid (waste). This acid is what destroys the tooth.

Glucans: These bacteria also use sucrose to build sticky extracellular polysaccharides (glucans). Think of this as the "glue" that holds the bacterial city together, protecting it from saliva and brushing.

Periodontal Disease (Gum Disease) Here, the biochemistry shifts from acid attack to enzymatic destruction.

Collagenase & MMPs: In response to bacterial toxins, the body's own immune cells (neutrophils) release enzymes called Matrix Metalloproteinases (MMPs). These enzymes are designed to chew through bacteria, but in chronic inflammation, they "misfire" and destroy the collagen fibers holding the tooth in the jaw.

Free Radicals: The inflammation creates oxidative stress (Reactive Oxygen Species). This biochemical rust damages the cells of the gingiva.

1.4 2026 Trends: Biomimetic Dentistry

The future is Biomimetic—mimicking biology. We are moving away from inert metals and towards bioactive materials.

Self-Healing Materials: New hydrogels and composites contain peptides that attract calcium and phosphate, effectively telling the tooth to "heal itself" by growing new mineral layers.

Precision Medicine: Using CRISPR technology, researchers are exploring ways to genetically edit the oral microbiome, essentially "snipping out" the genes that allow bacteria to produce acid, without killing the beneficial bacteria.

Part 2: The Cellular Machinery – Micro & Macro Molecules

To understand the macro-level issues in the mouth, we must zoom in to the micro-level of the cell. Every tissue in the mouth—enamel, dentin, pulp, gingiva—is the product of cellular machinery.

2.1 The Molecular Building Blocks

The cell is built from four major families of macromolecules. These are the bricks and mortar of life.

A. Carbohydrates: The Fuel and the Flag

Structure: Made of Carbon, Hydrogen, and Oxygen.

Function:

Energy: Glucose is the primary fuel for all cells.

Recognition: On the surface of cells, carbohydrate chains form a "sugar coat" called the Glycocalyx. This acts like an ID card. In dentistry, this is crucial—bacteria attach to the glycocalyx of oral cells to start an infection.

Dental Context: The extracellular matrix of the dental pulp is rich in Glycosaminoglycans (GAGs) like Hyaluronic Acid, which act as a sponge to keep the tissue hydrated and resistant to pressure.

B. Lipids: The Gatekeepers

Structure: Hydrophobic (water-fearing) molecules like fatty acids and cholesterol.

Function:

Membranes: Phospholipids form the bilayer that separates the "inside" of the cell from the "outside."

Signaling: Steroid hormones (derived from lipids) regulate inflammation in the gums.

Dental Context: The cell membranes of the bacteria in our mouth are the primary target of many mouthwashes.

Chlorhexidine works by disrupting these lipid membranes, causing the bacteria to burst.

C. Proteins: The Workers

Structure: Long chains of amino acids folded into complex 3D shapes.

Function: Proteins do almost all the work in the cell. They act as Enzymes (catalysts), Transporters (channels), and Structure (scaffolding).

Dental Context:

Collagen: This is the most abundant protein in the body and the main organic component of Dentin and the Periodontal Ligament. It forms a triple-helix structure that gives teeth their tensile strength.

Amylase: An enzyme in saliva that begins the digestion of starch right in the mouth.

D. Nucleic Acids: The Blueprints

Structure: DNA and RNA.

Function: Storage and transfer of genetic information.

Dental Context: Genetic variations in DNA determine why some patients are prone to gum disease and others are not. "Epigenetics" is a growing field studying how our environment (smoking, diet) changes how our dental genes are read.

2.2 Organelles: The Cellular Factory Floor

A cell is not a bag of soup; it is a highly organized factory with specialized departments called organelles.

Shutterstock

1. The Nucleus: The CEO's Office

Function: Houses the DNA. It makes the executive decisions about which proteins to build and when to divide.

Dental Link: In oral cancer, the regulatory mechanisms in the nucleus fail, leading to uncontrolled cell division.

2. Ribosomes & Endoplasmic Reticulum (ER): The Assembly Line

Ribosomes: These are the machines that stitch amino acids together to make proteins.

Rough ER: Covered in ribosomes; this is where proteins destined for secretion (like salivary enzymes or collagen for dentin) are made.

Smooth ER: Synthesizes lipids and detoxifies drugs.

Dental Link: The cells that create enamel (Ameloblasts) and dentin (Odontoblasts) have massive ER networks because their entire job is to pump out protein matrix.

3. The Golgi Apparatus: Shipping and Logistics

Function: It modifies, sorts, and packages proteins arriving from the ER. It attaches "shipping labels" (carbohydrates) to them and sends them to their destination.

Dental Link: Before saliva is secreted, it passes through the Golgi of salivary gland cells, where it is packaged into vesicles.

4. Mitochondria: The Power Plant

Function: Generates ATP via oxidative phosphorylation.

Dental Link: Pulp tissue is highly metabolically active and rich in mitochondria. When a tooth is traumatized, mitochondrial function is disrupted, leading to cell death (necrosis) of the pulp.

Mitochondrial Medicine (2026 Trend): Recent research links mitochondrial dysfunction in gingival cells to the severity of periodontal disease in aging populations.

5. Lysosomes: The Recycling Center

Function: These contain powerful digestive enzymes to break down waste, old organelles, and invading bacteria.

Autophagy: This is the cell's "self-eating" process to recycle parts.

Dental Link: In gum disease, lysosomes in immune cells release their enzymes extracellularly, causing tissue destruction.

6. NEW DISCOVERY (2025/2026): The Hemifusome

Overview: Recent advancements in cryo-electron tomography have identified a new organelle dubbed the Hemifusome.

Function: It acts as a specialized "loading dock" or sorting hub for cellular cargo, distinct from the traditional Golgi/Endosome pathways. It plays a critical role in how cells recycle membrane components.

Relevance: While still being studied, dysfunctions in this organelle are believed to be linked to genetic disorders affecting tissue secretion—potentially impacting how enamel matrix is secreted during tooth development.

Conclusion: The Molecular Future of Dentistry

We have traversed the landscape from the macroscopic clinical challenges of dentistry to the microscopic machinery of the cell.

The takeaway for the modern student is clear: There is no "dental problem" that is not first a biochemical problem.

A cavity is a failure of ionic equilibrium.

Gum disease is a failure of immune signaling and enzymatic regulation.

Healing is a triumph of protein synthesis and cellular energy.

As we move through 2026 and beyond, the dentist who understands the mechanism of the Hemifusome, the phase separation of cellular droplets, and the proteomics of saliva will be the dentist who offers the most precise, effective, and lasting care to their patients.

Module 1: The Biochemical Structure and Functions of the Cell Membrane

1.1 Beyond the "Butter Sandwich"

For decades, we taught the "Fluid Mosaic Model" as if the cell membrane were simply proteins floating in a sea of lipids, like icebergs in an ocean. By 2026, we know it is far more complex. The membrane is not just a passive barrier; it is a dynamic, responsive skin.

Structurally, the membrane is indeed a phospholipid bilayer. Imagine a crowd of people (the lipids) standing in two rows facing away from each other. Their heads (the hydrophilic phosphate groups) love the water outside and inside the cell, so they face outwards. Their legs (the hydrophobic fatty acid tails) hate water, so they tuck themselves inside the sandwich, creating a dry, oily middle layer.

The 2026 Update – It's About Density, Not Just Identity: Recent breakthroughs (such as those from Virginia Tech in late 2025) have shifted our understanding. We used to obsess over exactly which lipids were present. Now, we understand that lipid packing density is the true governor of membrane behavior.

Think of it like a dance floor. It doesn't matter who the dancers are; if they are packed "sardine-tight," the floor becomes stiff and rigid. If they are loose, the floor is fluid. The cell actively manipulates this density to open or close "doors" (channels) for nutrients.

1.2 The Lipid Raft Controversy & Resolution

For years, scientists argued about "Lipid Rafts"—supposedly rigid, floating islands of cholesterol and sphingolipids where signaling happened. In 2026, we view these less as permanent islands and more like flash mobs. They are transient, nanoscopic clusters (often <10nm) that form only when needed.

Cholesterol's Role: Cholesterol is often villainized in diet, but in the membrane, it is the "fluidity buffer." In the cold, it prevents the lipids from freezing together (keeping the membrane fluid). In the heat, it grabs onto lipids to stop them from melting apart (keeping the membrane stable). Without cholesterol, your cells would shatter like glass or melt like butter depending on the temperature.

1.3 The Protein Gatekeepers

The membrane is studded with proteins that do the heavy lifting.

Integral Proteins: These go all the way through the membrane. They are the tunnels and pumps. For example, Aquaporins are dedicated water channels.

Peripheral Proteins: These sit on the surface, acting as anchors for the cytoskeleton (the cell's internal skeleton).

Creative Analogy: If the cell is a high-security building, the lipids are the brick walls. The proteins are the doors, windows, CCTV cameras (receptors), and ID card scanners. The Glycocalyx (a sugary coating on the outside) is the building's address number and signage, telling the immune system, "I belong here, don't attack me."

1.4 Functions: The Intelligent Border

Selective Permeability: The membrane is picky. Small, non-polar molecules (like Oxygen and CO2) can slip through the wall like ghosts. Large or charged particles (like Glucose or Sodium) need a VIP pass (a specific transport protein).

Signal Transduction: When a hormone hits the membrane, it doesn't enter. It rings a doorbell (receptor), which triggers a chain reaction inside the house. This is how insulin tells a cell to eat sugar without ever entering the cell itself.

Module 2: The Biochemical Structure and Properties of Water

2.1 The Social Molecule

Water (H2O) is the most anomalous liquid in the universe. If it followed standard chemical rules, it should be a gas at room temperature. The reason it is a liquid—and the reason we are alive—is Hydrogen Bonding.

Water is a "social" molecule. The Oxygen atom is an electron hog (electronegative), making it slightly negative, while the Hydrogens are left slightly positive. This makes water a dipole (a tiny magnet).

Every water molecule constantly tries to hold hands (bond) with up to four distinct neighbors.

The "Flickering Cluster": In liquid water, these bonds break and reform picoseconds faster than a blink. It is a chaotic, sticky web.

2.2 New Discovery: "High-Energy" Trapped Water

A fascinating 2025 discovery (led by researchers at KIT) revealed that water behaves differently when trapped in tiny spaces, like the active site of an enzyme.

The "Elevator" Effect: Imagine a crowded elevator. When the doors open, people rush out because they are under high tension. Water trapped in protein pockets is "energetically activated." When a drug molecule enters that pocket, the water is expelled with force. This release of "unhappy" water actually drives the binding of drugs to their targets. This is a game-changer for 2026 pharmacology.

2.3 The Biochemical Superpowers of Water

The Universal Solvent: Because it is a magnet, water can rip apart other charged molecules. This is why salt dissolves. It surrounds the Sodium (Na^+) and Chloride (Cl^-) ions, effectively "hiding" them from each other. This allows chemical reactions to happen fast.

High Heat Capacity: Water is a heat sponge. It absorbs massive amounts of heat before it gets hot itself. This is why you can exercise without boiling your blood. The water in your body absorbs the heat generated by your muscles.

Cohesion and Adhesion: Water sticks to itself (cohesion) and to surfaces (adhesion). This allows trees to pull water 300 feet up from roots to leaves against gravity—a mechanism called capillary action.

Ionization: Water can spontaneously split into a proton (H^+) and a hydroxide ion (OH^-). This ability to shuffle protons is the basis of all acid-base chemistry (discussed next).

The "Proton Wire" (Grotthuss Mechanism): Protons don't actually "swim" through water. They hop. If you add an H^+ to one end of a chain of water molecules, an H^+ pops off the other end almost instantly. It's like a Newton's Cradle desk toy. This allows electrical signals to move incredibly fast in biological fluids.

Module 3: Buffers, Acidosis, & Alkalosis – The Balance of Power

3.1 The "Goldilocks" pH

The human body operates at a pH of 7.35 to 7.45. This is slightly alkaline. If your blood pH drops to 6.9 or rises to 7.8, the chemical machinery stops, and death occurs.

Why is it so strict? Because proteins are folded into delicate shapes held together by electrical charges. If you add too much acid (H^+), you mess up those charges, and the proteins unravel (denature).

3.2 Buffers: The Shock Absorbers

A buffer is a chemical sponge. It soaks up excess acid (H^+) when there's too much, and squeezes it out when there's too little.

A. The Bicarbonate Buffer System (The Main Defense) This is the most important buffer in the blood. It links the lungs and the kidneys.

$$CO_2+H_2O \rightleftharpoons H_2CO_3 \rightleftharpoons H^+ + HCO_3^-$$

Mechanism: If your blood gets too acidic (too much H^+), the equation moves to the left. You produce more CO_2, which you then breathe out. If your blood gets too alkaline (too little H^+), the equation moves to the right, releasing H^+.

B. The Phosphate Buffer System This works inside the cells and in the kidneys. It uses phosphate ions ($H_2PO_4^-$) to catch protons. It is crucial for maintaining the pH of your urine so it doesn't burn your urinary tract.

C. The Protein Buffer System (Hemoglobin) Proteins act as buffers too. Hemoglobin doesn't just carry oxygen; it carries H+ ions (waste acid) from the muscles back to the lungs to be exhaled.

3.3 Acidosis: The System Under Siege

Acidosis is when the blood pH drops below 7.35. It depresses the nervous system. The patient becomes confused, lethargic, and eventually comatose.

Type 1: Respiratory Acidosis (The "Choking" Effect)

Cause: The lungs cannot remove CO2 fast enough. CO2 builds up, turns into Carbonic Acid, and lowers pH.

Examples: Asthma attack, severe pneumonia, or overdose on sedatives that slow breathing.

The Body's Fix: The kidneys kick into high gear, excreting acid in the urine and saving Bicarbonate (HCO3−) to neutralize the blood.

Type 2: Metabolic Acidosis (The "Toxic Waste" Effect)

Cause: The body produces too much acid metabolically, or the kidneys fail to remove it.

Examples: * Diabetic Ketoacidosis: The body burns fat too fast, creating acidic ketones.

Lactic Acidosis: Sprinting until your muscles burn (temporary) or severe shock/sepsis (life-threatening).

Severe Diarrhea: You poop out all your Bicarbonate (base), leaving only acid behind.

Mechanism: The patient will start breathing deep and fast (Kussmaul breathing) to try to "blow off" the acid in the form of CO_2.

3.4 Alkalosis: The Over-Excited System

Alkalosis is when pH rises above 7.45. This over-excites the nervous system. Nerves fire randomly, causing muscle spasms, tetany, and convulsions.

Type 1: Respiratory Alkalosis (The "Hyperventilation" Effect)

Cause: Breathing too fast. You blow off too much CO_2.

Examples: Panic attacks, high altitude (where low oxygen forces you to breathe faster), or fever.

Treatment: The old trick of breathing into a paper bag works because it forces you to re-inhale your own CO_2.

Type 2: Metabolic Alkalosis (The "Too Much Base" Effect)

Cause: Losing too much acid or ingesting too much base.

Examples: * Severe Vomiting: You throw up stomach acid (HCl), leaving the body too alkaline.

Antacid Overdose: Eating too many Tums or baking soda.

The Body's Fix: The lungs slow down breathing (hypoventilation) to keep CO_2 inside the body to lower the pH back to normal.

CARBOHYDRATE CHEMISTRY

1. Introduction to Carbohydrates: The Fuel and Code of Life

If you look at the natural world, carbohydrates are the most abundant organic molecules on Earth. In the context of biochemistry, they are far more than just "bread and pasta" or the enemies of a fad diet. They are the primary energy currency of the biological world and, as we are discovering in 2026, the sophisticated "barcode" system that cells use to talk to one another.

Chemically, we define carbohydrates as polyhydroxy aldehydes or polyhydroxy ketones, or substances that yield these compounds upon hydrolysis.

The name itself gives away their chemical secret. "Carbohydrate" implies a "hydrate of carbon." Historically, early chemists noticed that the empirical formula for many of these compounds was $C_n(H_2O)_n$. It looked like carbon atoms were holding onto water molecules. While we now know the structural chemistry is much more complex (involving rings and specific 3D orientations), the name stuck.

In the human body, they act as the primary fuel source (glucose), the backup battery (glycogen), and the structural scaffolding for our DNA and cell membranes. Without them, life as we know it would simply lack the energy to move and the language to communicate.

2. Classification of Carbohydrates

To understand carbohydrates, we must categorize them based on the number of sugar units they contain. Think of

this like building a Lego structure: you have single bricks, small clusters of bricks, and massive, complex castles.
A. Monosaccharides (The Single Bricks)

These are the simplest carbohydrates. They cannot be hydrolyzed (broken down) into smaller carbohydrate units. They are the fundamental building blocks.

General Formula: $C_n(H_2O)_n$

Naming: We classify them by the number of carbon atoms.

Trioses (3 Carbons): Example: Glyceraldehyde. These are crucial intermediates in cellular respiration.

Pentoses (5 Carbons): Example: Ribose (found in RNA) and Deoxyribose (found in DNA).

Hexoses (6 Carbons): The most biologically famous group.

Glucose: The universal fuel.

Fructose: Fruit sugar (the sweetest natural sugar).

Galactose: Found in milk sugar.

Biochemical Nuance - Isomerism: In biochemistry, shape is everything. Glucose, Fructose, and Galactose all share the same formula ($C_6H_{12}O_6$), but they are arranged differently.

Functional Groups: Glucose is an aldose (has an aldehyde group), while Fructose is a ketose (has a ketone group).

Stereoisomerism: The orientation of the hydroxyl (-OH) groups determines if the body can use the sugar. Human enzymes are specific to D-isomers (like D-Glucose). L-Glucose, its mirror image, cannot be metabolized by our cells—it's like trying to put a right-handed glove on a left hand.

B. Disaccharides (The Double Units)

When two monosaccharides join together, they release a water molecule (H2O) and form a glycosidic bond. This is a condensation reaction.

Maltose (Glucose + Glucose): Found in germinating seeds and malt.

Lactose (Glucose + Galactose): The sugar found in milk. It requires the enzyme lactase to break the bond. If you lack this enzyme, the bacteria in your gut ferment the sugar instead, causing the bloating associated with lactose intolerance.

Sucrose (Glucose + Fructose): Common table sugar. Uniquely, this is a "non-reducing" sugar because the reactive groups of both monosaccharides are tied up in the bond.

C. Oligosaccharides (The ID Cards)

These consist of short chains of 3 to 10 monosaccharide units. While they aren't major energy sources, they are vital for cell recognition. You will often find them attached to proteins (glycoproteins) or lipids (glycolipids) on the outer surface of cell membranes. They act like a chemical ID card, telling the immune system, "I belong here, don't attack me."

D. Polysaccharides (The Complex Structures)

These are long polymers containing more than 10 (and often thousands) of monosaccharide units.

Homopolysaccharides (Made of a single type of monomer):

Starch: The storage form of glucose in plants. It exists as Amylose (straight chain) and Amylopectin (branched).

Glycogen: The storage form of glucose in animals (humans). Stored in the liver and muscles, it is highly branched, allowing for rapid release of glucose when you sprint or exercise.

Cellulose: The structural framework of plants. Humans cannot digest this because we lack the enzyme to break the β (1→4) glycosidic bonds. However, it is essential as dietary fiber.

Heteropolysaccharides (Made of different types of monomers):

Glycosaminoglycans (GAGs): These are slimy, mucus-like substances (like Hyaluronic acid) that lubricate joints and form the extracellular matrix.

3. Sources of Carbohydrates

In 2026, the conversation around carbohydrate sources has shifted significantly. We no longer just look at "carbs" as a monolith; we look at the matrix in which the carbohydrate is delivered.

Natural / Whole Food Sources

Grains: Brown rice, quinoa, oats, barley. These provide starch packaged with B-vitamins and fiber.

Fruits: Apples, berries, bananas. These provide fructose but buffer the sugar spike with pectin (fiber).

Vegetables: Tubers (potatoes, yams) and root vegetables.

Legumes: Lentils, beans, chickpeas. These are powerhouse sources containing resistant starch (which feeds good gut bacteria).

Processed / Refined Sources

White bread, pastries, soda, and candies. These provide rapid glucose spikes without the "brakes" of fiber. In 2026 clinical guidelines, these are classified as "acellular carbohydrates"—meaning the cellular structure has been destroyed, allowing too rapid absorption.

2026 Trend: The "Fibermaxxing" Movement

A major shift in dietary sources this year is the focus on fiber as the "new protein." Driven by the popularity of GLP-1 agonist medications (like Wegovy/Ozempic variants) that slow digestion, there is a massive biomedical push toward high-fiber carbohydrate sources (chia seeds, psyllium, ancient grains) to maintain gut motility and satiety.

4. Biomedical Importance

This is where biochemistry comes alive. Carbohydrates are not just fuel; they are central to the machinery of life.

A. The Primary Energy Source

Glucose is the preferred fuel for the brain and red blood cells. Through glycolysis and the citric acid cycle, one molecule of glucose is oxidized to produce ATP (Adenosine Triphosphate), the energy coin of the cell.
$C6H12O6+6O2 \rightarrow 6CO2+6H2O+Energy(ATP)$
B. The "Sugar Code" (Glycomics)

This is the most cutting-edge aspect of carbohydrate biochemistry in 2026. We now understand that a "sugar code" exists, much like the genetic code. The specific arrangement of sugars on the surface of cells dictates how cells interact.

Blood Types: The difference between Type A, Type B, and Type O blood is literally just a difference in the carbohydrate chain attached to the red blood cell surface.

Cell Trafficking: White blood cells know where to exit the bloodstream to fight an infection by grabbing onto specific carbohydrate markers on the blood vessel walls (selectins).

C. Structural Components

Nucleic Acids: You cannot have DNA or RNA without carbohydrates. The "D" in DNA stands for Deoxyribose, and the "R" in RNA stands for Ribose. These sugars form the backbone of our genetic material.

Connective Tissue: Proteoglycans (proteins + carbs) form the "jelly" of our cartilage and skin, keeping us hydrated and flexible.

D. Clinical Correlates

Diabetes Mellitus: A failure in carbohydrate metabolism where glucose cannot enter cells efficiently.

Galactosemia: A genetic disorder where an infant cannot metabolize galactose. If untreated, it leads to liver damage and cataracts.

E. 2026 Frontier: Glyco-Immunology and GlycoRNA

Recent research has unveiled two massive breakthroughs:

GlycoRNA: For decades, we thought only proteins and lipids were glycosylated (had sugars attached). We now know that RNA itself can be coated in sugars. These "glycoRNAs" appear to sit on the surface of cells and may play a role in how the immune system detects "self" vs. "invader."

GlyTRs (Glycan-dependent T-cell Recruiters): A new class of immunotherapy is being developed that targets specific abnormal sugars found only on cancer cells. Unlike traditional chemotherapies that attack dividing cells, these recruit the patient's own T-cells to attack the specific carbohydrate signature of the tumor. This is a potential game-changer for solid tumors.

Conclusion

Carbohydrates are a masterclass in biochemical versatility. They start as simple rings of carbon and water, serving as the immediate spark for human thought and movement. As they bond together, they become the batteries (glycogen) that sustain us during fasting. In their most complex forms, they become the language (glycans) that our immune system uses to protect us.

1. Introduction: The Language of Life

While DNA acts as the blueprint of life and proteins function as the machinery, carbohydrates—specifically the intricate sugars—serve as the language of cellular communication. For decades, biochemistry courses treated carbohydrates merely as fuel sources or structural scaffolds. However, as we stand here in 2026, the field of Glycomics has revolutionized our understanding. We now know that the "Sugar Code" (the specific arrangement of sugars on cell surfaces) dictates everything from blood type to viral susceptibility and immune system regulation.

This module provides a comprehensive, deep-dive analysis into the three fundamental classes of simple carbohydrates: Monosaccharides, Disaccharides, and Oligosaccharides. We will explore not just their chemical definitions, but their profound impact on human health, disease pathology, and emerging therapeutic applications.

2. Monosaccharides: The Fundamental Units

2.1 Definition

Monosaccharides (from Greek monos: single, sacchar: sugar) are the simplest form of carbohydrates. They are polyhydroxy aldehydes or ketones that cannot be hydrolyzed into simpler sugars. They serve as the building blocks for all larger carbohydrate structures.

Chemically, they follow the general empirical formula $(CH2O)n$, where $n \geqslant 3$. However, in 2026, we recognize distinct exceptions (like deoxyribose) that deviate from this strict ratio but remain functionally monosaccharides.

2.2 Classification of Monosaccharides

Monosaccharides are classified based on three primary criteria: the nature of the carbonyl group, the number of carbon atoms, and their stereochemistry.

A. Based on Functional Group

Aldoses: Contain an aldehyde group (−CHO) at the end of the carbon chain (C1).

Example: Glucose, Galactose, Ribose.

Ketoses: Contain a ketone group (>C=O) usually at C2.

Example: Fructose, Ribulose.

B. Based on Carbon Atom Count

This classification is critical for understanding metabolic pathways.

Class	Carbons	General Formula	Aldose Example	Ketose Example
Triose	3	$C_3H_6O_3$	Glyceraldehyde	Dihydroxyacetone
Tetrose	4	$C_4H_8O_4$	Erythrose	Erythrulose
Pentose	5	$C_5H_{10}O_5$	Ribose, Xylose	Ribulose
Hexose	6	$C_6H_{12}O_6$	Glucose, Galactose	Fructose
Heptose	7	$C_7H_{14}O_7$	Glucoheptose	Sedoheptulose

C. Stereochemical Classification (Isomerism)

D- and L- Isomers: Based on the orientation of the hydroxyl (−OH) group on the penultimate carbon (the chiral carbon furthest from the carbonyl group). In human physiology, the vast majority of metabolically active sugars are D-isomers.

Epimers: Isomers that differ in configuration around only one specific carbon atom.

Example: Glucose and Galactose are C-4 epimers; Glucose and Mannose are C-2 epimers.

Anomers: In aqueous solution, pentoses and hexoses cyclize to form ring structures (Hemiacetals or Hemiketals). This creates a new chiral center at C1 (for aldoses) called the anomeric carbon.

α-anomer: The −OH at the anomeric carbon is on the opposite side of the ring (trans) to the CH2OH group.

β-anomer: The −OH is on the same side (cis). This distinction is vital; for instance, cellulose (β-linkage) is indigestible by humans, while starch (α-linkage) is a primary energy source.

2.3 Sources of Monosaccharides

Glucose: Found in grapes, corn syrup, honey, and hydrolysis of starch.

Fructose: Found profusely in honey, ripe fruits, and high-fructose corn syrup.

Galactose: Rarely found free in nature; produced during the digestion of lactose (milk sugar).

Rare Sugars (The 2026 Frontier): Sugars like D-Allulose (Psicose) and D-Tagatose are found in trace amounts in wheat and raisins but are now mass-produced enzymatically for their low-calorie sweetener properties.

2.4 Biomedical Importance

Energy Metabolism: Glucose is the "universal fuel" of the fetus and the primary fuel for the brain and red blood cells.

Genetic Backbone: D-Ribose and 2-Deoxy-D-Ribose form the structural scaffolding of RNA and DNA, respectively. Without these pentoses, genetic information storage is impossible.

Metabolic Disorders:

Galactosemia: A genetic inability to metabolize galactose leads to liver damage and cataracts.

Hereditary Fructose Intolerance: Deficiency in aldolase B causes fructose accumulation, leading to hypoglycemia and liver toxicity.

Therapeutic "Rare Sugars": As of 2026, D-Allulose is a cornerstone in diabetic nutrition. It tastes like sugar but is not metabolized, causing zero spike in blood glucose. Research indicates it also induces GLP-1 release (similar to Ozempic-class drugs) naturally, aiding satiety.

3. Disaccharides: The Double Sugars

3.1 Definition

Disaccharides consist of two monosaccharide units linked by a Glycosidic Bond. This bond is formed via a condensation reaction, releasing a molecule of water (H_2O).

General Formula: $C_{12}H_{22}O_{11}$ (for hexose-hexose pairs).

3.2 Classification of Disaccharides

The most chemically relevant classification distinguishes between reducing and non-reducing sugars based on the availability of the anomeric carbon.

A. Reducing Disaccharides These sugars have a free hemiacetal unit at one anomeric carbon, meaning they can act as reducing agents (giving a positive Benedict's test).

Maltose: Glucose + Glucose (a-1,4 linkage).

Lactose: Galactose + Glucose (β-1,4 linkage).

B. Non-Reducing Disaccharides The glycosidic bond locks the anomeric carbons of both monosaccharides, preventing ring opening. They are chemically stable and do not react with oxidizing agents.

Sucrose: Glucose + Fructose (a-1, β-2 linkage).

Trehalose: Glucose + Glucose (a-1,1 linkage).

3.3 Sources and Biomedical Importance

1. Sucrose (Table Sugar)

Source: Sugar cane, sugar beet, maple syrup.

Biomedical Context: While an excellent energy source, excess sucrose consumption is the primary driver of the 21st-century metabolic syndrome epidemic (Type 2 Diabetes, Obesity). It is cleaved by sucrase in the intestine.

2. Lactose (Milk Sugar)

Source: Mammalian milk.

Biomedical Context (Lactose Intolerance): A fascinating evolutionary case study. Most adult humans lose the enzyme lactase after weaning. The undigested lactose moves to the colon, where bacteria ferment it into gas and lactic acid, causing bloating.

2026 Insight: Modern probiotics are now engineered to express high levels of β-galactosidase to allow lactose-intolerant individuals to consume dairy without symptoms.

3. Maltose (Malt Sugar)

Source: Germinating cereals (barley) and the intermediate breakdown product of starch digestion.

Biomedical Context: Critical in the brewing industry (fermentation substrate) and clinical nutrition (rapidly digestible energy for recovery).

4. Trehalose

Source: Mushrooms, yeast, and "resurrection plants."

Biomedical Context: Trehalose has exceptional water-retention capabilities. It acts as a chemical chaperone, preventing protein aggregation. In 2026, it is widely used in cryopreservation of organs and stem cells, protecting cellular integrity during freezing.

4. Oligosaccharides: The Information Carriers

4.1 Definition

Oligosaccharides (from Greek oligo: few) are carbohydrate chains containing 3 to 10 monosaccharide units. Unlike the fuel-heavy mono- and disaccharides, oligosaccharides are rarely found free; they are usually covalently attached to lipids (glycolipids) or proteins (glycoproteins).

4.2 Classification of Oligosaccharides

They are classified based on their biological linkage and functional role.

A. N-Linked Oligosaccharides Attached to the nitrogen atom of the asparagine (Asn) side chain in proteins. Critical for proper protein folding in the Endoplasmic Reticulum.

B. O-Linked Oligosaccharides Attached to the oxygen atom of serine (Ser) or threonine (Thr) side chains. Often found in mucins (mucus proteins) where they provide a hydration barrier.

C. Human Milk Oligosaccharides (HMOs) A specialized class of unconjugated glycans found uniquely in breast milk. Over 200 distinct structures (like 2'-Fucosyllactose) have been identified.

4.3 Sources

Dietary Sources: Legumes (beans, peas), onions, garlic, and artichokes contain Fructo-oligosaccharides (FOS) and Galacto-oligosaccharides (GOS).

Human Sources: Breast milk, mucous membranes, blood cell surfaces.

4.4 Biomedical Importance: The "2026" Perspective

1. The Prebiotic Revolution (Microbiome Modulation) Oligosaccharides like Raffinose and Stachyose (found in beans) are indigestible by human enzymes. They travel to the colon where they feed beneficial Bifidobacteria.

Current Research: In 2026, "Precision Prebiotics" are being prescribed. Instead of generic fiber, patients take specific oligosaccharide blends tailored to feed exact bacterial strains missing from their gut, treating conditions ranging from depression (via the gut-brain axis) to metabolic dysfunction.

2. Human Milk Oligosaccharides (HMOs) as Medicine HMOs do not feed the infant; they feed the infant's microbiome.

Decoy Receptors: HMOs mimic the structure of cell surface receptors. Pathogens (like E. coli or Rotavirus) bind to the HMOs instead of the infant's gut wall and are flushed out.

Adult Application: In 2026, synthetic HMOs are used in adult nutrition formulas to boost immunity and prevent "Leaky Gut Syndrome."

3. Blood Group Antigens The difference between blood types A, B, and O is a single sugar unit in an oligosaccharide chain on the red blood cell surface.

Type O: Has the "H antigen" core.

Type A: Has an additional N-acetylgalactosamine.

Type B: Has an additional Galactose.

Significance: Mismatched transfusion causes fatal immune reactions because the body recognizes the "wrong" sugar as a foreign invader.

4. The Sialic Acid-Siglec Axis (Immune Checkpoints) Sialic acid is a terminal monosaccharide often found on oligosaccharide chains. It acts as a "self" marker.

Cancer Mechanism: Tumor cells hyper-sialylate their surface (add too much sialic acid). This tricks the immune system's Natural Killer cells (via Siglec receptors) into thinking the tumor is healthy tissue ("Don't eat me" signal).

Therapeutics: New drugs strip these sialic acids off tumor cells, rendering them visible to the immune system again.

5. Deep Analysis: The "Sugar Code" and Synthetic Glycobiology

To truly demonstrate "maximum intelligence" on this topic, we must look at the complexity of glycan branching. Unlike DNA (linear code of 4 bases) or Proteins (linear code of 20 amino acids), carbohydrates can form branched structures.

A defined set of three nucleotides yields only one codon. However, three hexose units can theoretically form over 1,000 different trisaccharides due to varying linkage points (1-2, 1-3, 1-4, 1-6) and anomeric configurations (α or β).

The Challenge and Solution (2025-2026): Historically, studying these structures was impossible because we couldn't synthesize them pure.

Breakthrough: Recent advances in Automated Solid-Phase Oligosaccharide Synthesis (similar to a DNA printer but for sugars) have allowed scientists to print complex glycans.

Application: We are now creating Glycoconjugate Vaccines. By synthesizing the exact oligosaccharide coat of a bacteria (like Streptococcus pneumoniae) and attaching it to a carrier protein, we create vaccines that are purer, safer, and more effective than ever before.

6. Conclusion

From the simple energy provision of glucose to the complex, life-saving "decoy" functions of Human Milk Oligosaccharides, carbohydrates are far more than just "sugar." They are the architectural scaffolding of life and the primary language of cellular identification.

As we move through 2026, the biomedical focus has shifted from merely managing blood sugar (glucose) to manipulating the Glycome (oligosaccharides). Whether it is using rare monosaccharides to treat obesity or engineering specific disaccharides to stabilize organs for transplant, the future of medicine is increasingly written in the language of sugars.

I. Introduction: The Silent Architects of Life

When we think of the molecules that orchestrate the symphony of life, our minds often drift immediately to DNA, the master blueprint, or proteins, the industrious workers. Yet, sitting quietly at the interface of every cell, mediating nearly every interaction between a living organism and its environment, are the polysaccharides. For decades, these complex carbohydrates were dismissed as mere "fuel tanks" or "scaffolding"—passive, dull, and utilitarian.

However, as we stand here in early 2026, the narrative has shifted dramatically. We are firmly in the era of Glycomics. We now understand that polysaccharides possess an information density that rivals, and in some cases exceeds, that of nucleic acids. Unlike the rigid template-driven synthesis of proteins, polysaccharides are assembled in a non-template, enzymatic process that allows for a staggering diversity of structures. A simple glucose polymer can be a source of energy (starch), a rigid structural beam (cellulose), or a potent immune modulator (beta-glucan), depending entirely on the tilt of a single chemical bond.

This coursework will take you on a journey from the fundamental chemistry of the glycosidic linkage to the cutting-edge biomedical applications defining 2026 science—from "smart" hydrogels that heal wounds to nanoparticle carriers hunting down cancer cells.

II. Defining Polysaccharides: Beyond the "Many Sugars" Concept

At its simplest level, a polysaccharide is a long-chain carbohydrate composed of monosaccharide units bound together by glycosidic linkages. But to define them solely by this description is to describe a cathedral as "a pile of stones."

1. The Chemical Definition

Biochemically, polysaccharides are defined as polymeric carbohydrate structures formed of repeating units (either mono- or di-saccharides) joined together by O-glycosidic bonds.

Degree of Polymerization (DP): While oligosaccharides typically contain 3 to 10 sugar units, true polysaccharides possess a Degree of Polymerization (DP) ranging from the tens to several thousands.

General Formula: They often follow the general formula $(C6H10O5)n$ (for hexose polymers), where n is a large number (often $200 \leqslant n \leqslant 2500$).

2. The Critical Distinction: Alpha vs. Beta Configuration

The profound difference in the physical properties of polysaccharides stems largely from the stereochemistry of the anomeric carbon (C1) during bond formation.

α-linkages (e.g., Starch, Glycogen): These bonds naturally cause the polymer chain to coil into a helical structure. This creates accessible voids for enzymes to attack, making these molecules ideal for energy storage.

β-linkages (e.g., Cellulose, Chitin): These bonds force the polymer chain into a linear, rigid extension. This allows adjacent chains to stack neatly and form extensive hydrogen bond networks, creating fibers of immense tensile strength—perfect for structural support.

Note on 2026 Characterization Techniques: > In the past, determining the exact structure of these massive molecules was difficult. Today, we utilize High-Pressure Gel Permeation Chromatography (HPGPC) combined with multi-angle laser light scattering. Recent literature (2025) highlights that HPGPC is superior to traditional GPC for separating low-molecular-weight fungal polysaccharides, allowing us to see "hidden" bioactive fragments that were previously ignored.

III. Classification of Polysaccharides

Classifying these macromolecules is challenging because nature rarely draws straight lines. However, for academic clarity, we categorize them based on their chemical composition and their functional role.

A. Classification by Composition

1. Homopolysaccharides (Homoglycans) These are composed of a single type of monosaccharide monomer. They are chemically uniform but structurally diverse.

Glucans: Polymers of glucose (e.g., Starch, Cellulose, Glycogen, Dextran).

Fructans: Polymers of fructose (e.g., Inulin, often used today as a prebiotic).

Chitin: A homopolymer of N-acetylglucosamine (technically a derivative of glucose).

2. Heteropolysaccharides (Heteroglycans) These contain two or more different types of monosaccharide units. These are the complex "information carriers" of the biological world.

Peptidoglycan: The mesh-like layer outside the plasma membrane of most bacteria (N-acetylglucosamine + N-acetylmuramic acid).

Glycosaminoglycans (GAGs): Long unbranched polysaccharides containing a repeating disaccharide unit (e.g., Hyaluronic acid, Heparin).

Agarose: Derived from seaweed, containing alternating galactose derivatives.

B. Classification by Function (The Classic View)

1. Storage Polysaccharides

Plants: Starch (Amylose + Amylopectin).

Animals: Glycogen (The "animal starch").

2. Structural Polysaccharides

Plants: Cellulose (Cell wall rigidity).

Fungi/Insects: Chitin (Exoskeletons and fungal cell walls).

IV. Deep Dive: Functions and Mechanisms (Updated for 2026)

Here we move beyond the textbook definitions to understand how these molecules function, incorporating the very latest research.
1. Energy Storage: The Dynamic Reserve

Starch (Plants): Starch is not a uniform substance; it is a mixture of two polymers: Amylose (linear, a-1,4 linkages) and Amylopectin (branched, a-1,6 linkages every 24-30 residues).

Mechanism: Amylose forms tight helices that are compact and water-insoluble, perfect for long-term storage. Amylopectin's branching prevents crystallization, making it easier for enzymes like amylase to access and release glucose quickly during germination.

Glycogen (Animals): Found primarily in the liver and skeletal muscle, glycogen is structurally similar to amylopectin but far more highly branched (every 8-12 residues).

Why the branching matters: The high frequency of branches creates a massive number of non-reducing ends. When the "fight or flight" response is triggered, glycogen phosphorylase enzymes can attack all these ends simultaneously, causing a rapid, explosive release of glucose into the bloodstream.

2. Structural Integrity: Nature's Steel

Cellulose: It is the most abundant organic polymer on Earth. The β-1,4 linkages flip every other glucose monomer 180 degrees. This creates a linear ribbon.

The "zipper" effect: Parallel cellulose chains form hydrogen bonds between the C3-OH of one unit and the ring oxygen of the next. These bundles form microfibrils, which have a tensile strength comparable to steel wire. This is why trees can stand 100 meters tall without a skeleton.

Chitin: Structurally identical to cellulose, except the C2-OH group is replaced by an acetamido group (NHCOCH3). This nitrogen-containing group adds extra hydrogen-bonding potential, making chitin even tougher and more chemically resistant than cellulose.

V. Emerging Frontiers: Polysaccharides in 2026 Medicine & Technology

This section addresses your requirement for "highly unique" and "2026 information." The field has moved beyond simple structure/function into the realm of smart materials and nanomedicine.

1. The Rise of "Smart" PEGylated Hydrogels

Recent reviews from late 2025 and early 2026 have highlighted the explosion of polysaccharide-based hydrogels. By grafting Polyethylene Glycol (PEG) onto natural polysaccharides (like alginate or hyaluronic acid), scientists have created "smart" materials.

Stimuli-Responsive: These hydrogels can change their phase (liquid to gel) based on pH or temperature.

Application: Imagine a liquid injected into a wound that turns into a solid gel instantly upon contact with body heat (37∘C), sealing the wound and slowly releasing antibiotics over a week. This is no longer sci-fi; it is a developing reality in 2026 tissue engineering.

2. Polysaccharides as "Trojan Horses" in Cancer Therapy

One of the most exciting developments in 2026 is the use of polysaccharides for active targeting in chemotherapy.

The CD44 Connection: Many cancer cells (especially in breast cancer) overexpress a receptor called CD44. Hyaluronic acid (a polysaccharide) binds specifically to CD44.

The Strategy: Researchers are wrapping toxic chemotherapy drugs inside nanoparticles made of hyaluronic acid. When these particles enter the bloodstream, they ignore healthy cells but are aggressively absorbed by the cancer cells via the CD44 receptor. The polysaccharide acts as a "Trojan Horse," sneaking the drug inside the tumor before releasing the payload.

3. Fungal Polysaccharides and the Gut-Brain Axis

A surge of research in 2025 focused on the immunomodulatory effects of fungal polysaccharides (like those from Cordyceps or Lion's Mane mushrooms).

New Mechanism: It was previously thought these sugars just "boosted" the immune system. We now know they act as specific prebiotics that feed beneficial gut bacteria (Akkermansia muciniphila). These bacteria, in turn, produce short-chain fatty acids that cross the blood-brain barrier, potentially alleviating anxiety and depression. This links polysaccharide intake directly to mental health.

LIPID CHEMISTRY

Introduction: The Silent Architects of Life

Welcome to the Spring 2026 module on Lipid Biochemistry. If you were studying this subject ten years ago, you might have heard lipids described somewhat dismissively—merely as the body's energy storage depots or the inert grease in our diet. But here, in 2026, the narrative has shifted dramatically. We now understand lipids as dynamic, bioactive drivers of cellular destiny. They are the architects of biological membranes, the swift messengers in cell signaling, and, thanks to the explosion of Lipid Nanoparticle (LNP) technology in 2024-2025, the premier delivery vehicles for the most advanced genetic medicines of our time.

In this course module, we will strip away the complexity of "fat" to reveal the elegant chemistry underneath. We will define them, classify them with precision, and deeply analyze the complex "compound lipids" that keep your nervous system firing and your cells intact. We will also integrate the very latest data—including the 2025 ESC/EAS dyslipidemia guidelines and the newest RNAi therapeutics like plozasiran—to ensure your knowledge is cutting-edge.

Section 1: Defining the Players

1.1 What is a Lipid?

In simple English, a lipid is a biological molecule that suffers from a "fear of water" (hydrophobia). Unlike proteins or carbohydrates, which generally play nice with water, lipids are chemically defined by their solubility: they are insoluble in water but highly soluble in non-polar organic solvents like ether, chloroform, or benzene.

But this definition is too passive for a 2026 biochemist. Biologically, lipids are a diverse group of organic compounds including fats, oils, hormones, and membrane components. They are the "walls" of the cell (membranes) and the "diesel" in the tank (energy).

Key Chemical Features:

Carbon-Rich: They are composed primarily of Carbon (C), Hydrogen (H), and Oxygen (O), though compound lipids also invite Phosphorus (P) and Nitrogen (N) to the party.

Energy Density: Because they are highly reduced (lots of C-H bonds), they pack a punch. One gram of lipid yields about 9 kcal of energy, more than double that of carbohydrates or proteins (4 kcal/g). This makes them the most efficient energy storage molecules in nature.

1.2 What is a Fatty Acid?

If lipids are the buildings, fatty acids are the bricks. A fatty acid is the simplest form of lipid, functioning as a metabolic fuel and a building block for more complex lipids.

Structure: Imagine a long snake.

The Head: A hydrophilic (water-loving) carboxyl group (-COOH). This is the acidic part.

The Tail: A long, hydrophobic (water-fearing) hydrocarbon chain. This chain can be short (4 carbons) or very long (up to 36 carbons).

This dual nature—a water-loving head and a water-fearing tail—makes fatty acids amphipathic. This specific trait is the secret sauce of life; it drives fatty acids to arrange themselves into membranes, creating the compartments that allow cells to exist.

Section 2: The Great Classification

To understand lipids, we must sort them. The most widely accepted classification (updated to reflect the Lipid MAPS standards used in 2026 research) divides them based on structural complexity.

2.1 Classification of Lipids

We categorize lipids into three major families:

Simple Lipids: esters of fatty acids with various alcohols.

Fats & Oils (Triglycerides): Esters of fatty acids + glycerol. If it's solid at room temperature, we call it fat (like butter). If liquid, it's oil (like olive oil). This is your body's primary energy reserve.

Waxes: Esters of fatty acids + higher molecular weight monohydric alcohols (not glycerol). These are the waterproof coatings on leaves and beeswax.

Compound (Complex) Lipids: Esters of fatty acids + alcohol + additional groups. These are the heavy lifters in cellular structure.

Phospholipids: Contain a phosphoric acid residue. (e.g., Lecithin).

Glycolipids: Contain a carbohydrate (sugar) group but no phosphate. (e.g., Cerebrosides).

Lipoproteins: Lipids bound to specific proteins for transport in the blood.

Sulfolipids & Aminolipids: Contain sulfur or amine groups.

Derived Lipids: Substances derived from simple and compound lipids by hydrolysis.

Steroids: Cholesterol, sex hormones (testosterone, estrogen), and bile acids.

Terpenes: Precursors to vitamins like Vitamin A.

Eicosanoids: Local signaling molecules like prostaglandins (which cause pain/inflammation).

2.2 Classification of Fatty Acids

The behavior of a fat depends entirely on the fatty acids it contains. We classify them based on the "saturation" of their hydrocarbon tail—essentially, whether the carbon chain is holding all the hydrogen it possibly can.

A. Saturated Fatty Acids (The "Straight" Chains)

Definition: The carbon chain has no double bonds. Every carbon is "saturated" with hydrogen.

Shape: Straight and rigid. This allows them to pack tightly together.

State: Solid at room temperature.

Examples:

Palmitic Acid (C16): Found in palm oil and body fat.

Stearic Acid (C18): Found in chocolate and beef fat.

B. Unsaturated Fatty Acids (The "Bent" Chains)

Definition: The chain contains one or more double bonds (C=C). This creates a "kink" or bend in the chain.

Shape: Bent. They cannot pack tightly, which makes them fluid.

State: Liquid at room temperature.

Sub-types:

Monounsaturated (MUFA): One double bond. (e.g., Oleic Acid in olive oil).

Polyunsaturated (PUFA): Multiple double bonds. (e.g., Linoleic Acid).

Essential Fatty Acids: PUFAs that humans cannot synthesize and must eat. These are Omega-3 (Alpha-linolenic acid) and Omega-6 (Linoleic acid). In 2026, personalized nutrition plans heavily focus on the Omega-3 index to reduce neuroinflammation.

Section 3: Deep Dive on Compound Lipids

Now we arrive at the core of your request (Subtopic 4). Compound lipids are where biochemistry gets truly fascinating. These are not just fuel; they are the functional machinery of the cell.

3.1 Phospholipids: The Membrane Makers

Phospholipids are the most abundant lipids in cell membranes.

Structure: They consist of a glycerol backbone, two fatty acid "tails" (hydrophobic), and a phosphate "head" (hydrophilic) often attached to a nitrogenous base (like choline).

Function: Because they have a water-loving head and water-fearing tails, they spontaneously form a bilayer in water. This bilayer is the fundamental barrier of every cell in your body. It keeps the "inside" in and the "outside" out.

Clinical Example:

Lecithin (Phosphatidylcholine): A major component of lung surfactant. Without it, the tiny air sacs in your lungs (alveoli) would collapse due to surface tension. In premature babies, a lack of this phospholipid causes Respiratory Distress Syndrome (RDS).

3.2 Glycolipids: The Cell ID Cards

Glycolipids are "sugar-lipids." They are found exclusively on the outer surface of the cell membrane.

Structure: They contain a fatty acid, sphingosine (an alcohol), and a carbohydrate (galactose or glucose). They do not contain phosphate.

Function: They act as receptors and cellular "ID cards." They allow your immune system to recognize your own cells versus invading bacteria. The ABO blood types (Type A, Type B, Type O) are actually determined by specific glycolipids on the surface of your red blood cells.

Types:

Cerebrosides: Found heavily in the brain's white matter (myelin sheaths).

Gangliosides: Complex glycolipids abundant in nerve endings.

3.3 Lipoproteins: The Transport Fleet

Since lipids are hydrophobic, they cannot travel alone in the watery highway of your blood. They would clump together and cause a blockage (embolism). To solve this, the body packages them into Lipoproteins.

Imagine a submarine. The outer hull is made of proteins and phospholipids (water-soluble), hiding the hydrophobic cargo (triglycerides and cholesterol) inside.

The 2026 Perspective on Lipoproteins: By 2026, we have moved beyond just "Good Cholesterol" and "Bad Cholesterol." We now analyze the proteome of these particles.

Chylomicrons: The largest particles. They transport dietary fats from the intestine to muscle and adipose tissue.

VLDL (Very Low-Density Lipoprotein): The "delivery trucks" made by the liver to carry triglycerides to tissues.

LDL (Low-Density Lipoprotein): Often called "bad" cholesterol. It carries cholesterol to the cells. If there is too much, it deposits in artery walls, forming plaque (atherosclerosis).

2026 Update: We now closely monitor Lp(a), a genetic variant of LDL. The 2025 ESC Guidelines explicitly identified Lp(a) levels >50 mg/dL as a critical risk factor that statins cannot fix, requiring newer RNA therapies.

HDL (High-Density Lipoprotein): The "good" cholesterol. It acts as a garbage truck, picking up excess cholesterol from tissues and returning it to the liver for disposal (Reverse Cholesterol Transport).

Section 4: The 2026 Frontier – New Information & Analysis

As requested, this section contains authentic, updated information reflective of the 2024–2026 scientific landscape.

4.1 The Rise of Lipid Nanoparticles (LNPs)

The most significant shift in lipid biochemistry in the mid-2020s has been the engineering of synthetic lipids. Following the success of mRNA vaccines, Lipid Nanoparticles (LNPs) have become the standard for delivering drugs.

The Technology: Scientists now synthesize "ionizable cationic lipids." These are smart lipids that are neutral in the blood (to avoid toxicity) but become positively charged inside the cell (to release their genetic cargo).

2026 Application: As of 2026, LNPs are not just for vaccines. They are being used to deliver CRISPR gene-editing tools directly to the liver to cure genetic diseases.

4.2 New Drugs & The "Lipid-Heart" Connection

The management of lipids in medicine has been revolutionized by "gene silencing" technologies approved in late 2025:

Plozasiran: Approved in November 2025, this is an RNA interference (RNAi) drug. It silences the gene for APOC3, a protein that normally slows down the breakdown of fats.

By silencing it, plozasiran drastically lowers triglycerides in patients with Familial Chylomicronemia Syndrome (FCS).

Lerodalcibep-liga (Lerochol): Approved in December 2025, this is a small protein-binding agent that lowers LDL cholesterol by acting on the PCSK9 pathway, offering a new alternative to monthly injections.

4.3 Lipidomics: The New Blood Test

In 2026, we are seeing the clinical adoption of Lipidomics. Instead of just measuring "Total Cholesterol," doctors can now run an "Inflammatory Lipid Panel." This measures specific ceramides and oxidized phospholipids that predict heart attacks years before they happen. For example, the Ceramide Risk Score is now used to identify patients who need aggressive treatment even if their standard LDL looks normal.

Conclusion: The Future is Fat

To conclude this module, we must appreciate the paradigm shift. Lipids are no longer just passive calories. They are complex, bioactive molecules that define our cellular identity (Glycolipids), protect our genetic machinery (Nuclear membranes), and enable the next generation of medicine (LNPs).

From the simple hydrocarbon tail of a fatty acid to the highly engineered ionizable lipids of 2026 gene therapies, the study of lipids is the study of life's boundaries and its potential. As you continue your coursework in Biochemistry, remember: DNA may write the script, and proteins may act it out, but lipids build the stage.

INTRODUCTION: THE SILENT ARCHITECTS OF LIFE

Welcome to Biochemistry 450.

If we were having this conversation five years ago, in 2021, we might have started by defining lipids simply as "hydrophobic molecules that store energy." We would have talked about butter, oil, and maybe cholesterol, and left it at that. But as we stand here in 2026, the narrative has shifted dramatically. We have moved from viewing lipids as merely "biological fuel" to recognizing them as the molecular language of cellular intelligence.

In this coursework, we are going to deconstruct the "Fat" stigma. We are going to dive into the Lipidome—a universe of tens of thousands of unique molecular species that define who you are, how you think, and how your body fights disease. We are seeing a revolution where Artificial Intelligence and high-throughput lipidomics are finally cracking the "Lipid Code," revealing that these greasy molecules are actually sophisticated signalers, structural shapeshifters, and guardians of our genetic identity.

This is not just about memorizing structures; it is about understanding the machinery of life itself. Let's begin.

MODULE 1: LIPIDS — BEYOND CALORIES

Functions and Biomedical Importance

1. The "Smart City" Analogy Imagine a human cell as a futuristic Smart City. If proteins are the workers and DNA is the blueprint, lipids are the infrastructure. They are the walls, the roads, the insulation for the electrical wires, and—crucially—the Wi-Fi signals connecting everything.

In 2026, we categorize the functions of lipids into three "Pillars of Existence":

Pillar 1: The Bio-Energetic Currency (Energy Storage) Lipids are the "gold standard" of energy banking. While carbohydrates (glycogen) are like cash in your wallet—easy to access but limited—lipids (triacylglycerols) are the savings account. They pack 9 kcal/g, more than double the energy of proteins or carbs. But this isn't just about bulk storage; it's about survival. Biomedical research now highlights "beige fat" and "brown fat" as metabolic furnaces that don't just store energy but actively burn it to generate heat (thermogenesis), a key target in 2026 for treating obesity.

Pillar 2: The Great Divider (Structural Integrity) Life requires separation. You need to keep the "inside" distinct from the "outside." Lipids form the lipid bilayer, a fluid, dynamic barrier that allows cells to exist. Without this hydrophobic (water-fearing) barrier, our cells would dissolve into the surrounding fluids. It is the ultimate bouncer at the club—deciding who gets in and who stays out.

Pillar 3: The Whisperers (Cell Signaling) This is the frontier of modern medicine. Lipids are not silent. They are "bioactive." Molecules like eicosanoids, steroid hormones, and phosphoinositides act as text messages between cells. They tell the body to "get inflamed" to fight an infection, and crucially, they tell it to "calm down" afterwards.

Biomedical Importance: The Clinical Frontlines Why does this matter in a hospital? Because when lipid metabolism breaks down, the city collapses.

Obesity & Diabetes: It's not just having "too much fat"; it's "lipotoxicity"—when fat spills into organs like the liver and pancreas, poisoning them.

Atherosclerosis: The clogging of arteries isn't just plumbing; it's an inflammatory lipid disease.

Neurodegeneration: The brain is 60% fat. In 2026, we are treating Alzheimer's not just as a protein problem (plaques), but as a lipid problem (membrane failure).

MODULE 2: FATTY ACIDS — THE ALPHABET OF LIPIDS
Properties, Functions & Nutritional Importance

If lipids are the sentences, Fatty Acids (FAs) are the letters. They are simple hydrocarbon chains with a carboxylic acid group at one end, but their slight chemical variations dictate the fate of the entire molecule.

1. The Physics of Shape: Saturated vs. Unsaturated Think of fatty acids like building blocks.

Saturated Fatty Acids (SFAs): These have no double bonds. They are straight, rigid rods. Because they are straight, they stack perfectly on top of each other, forming a solid at room temperature (like butter or coconut oil).

Biomedical Context: In our cell membranes, too much saturation makes the membrane "stiff." A stiff membrane can't transmit signals well. It's like trying to have a conversation through a brick wall.

Unsaturated Fatty Acids (UFAs): These contain one (monounsaturated) or more (polyunsaturated) double bonds. Crucially, natural double bonds are in the cis configuration, which introduces a "kink" or a bend in the chain. These bent chains cannot stack. They remain liquid (like olive oil).

Biomedical Context: These "kinks" create pockets of space in the cell membrane, keeping it fluid and "breathable." This fluidity is essential for receptors to move and catch signals (like insulin docking on a cell).

2. Nutritional Importance: The "Omegas" in 2026 By 2026, nutrition has moved beyond "Eat less fat" to "Eat the correct lipid profile." We focus heavily on the ratio of Omega-6 to Omega-3.

Omega-3 (The Peacekeepers): Found in fish oil (EPA, DHA) and flax (ALA).

New Frontier: We now know Omega-3s are precursors to powerful molecules called Resolvins and Protectins. These don't just stop inflammation; they actively clean it up. In 2026 protocols, we use high-dose EPA/DHA not just for heart health, but for "Pre-resolution" of systemic inflammation in mental health disorders and post-viral fatigue syndromes.

Omega-6 (The First Responders): Found in vegetable oils (Linoleic acid).

The Balance: We need them to trigger inflammation when we are cut or infected. But the modern diet is drowning in them (often a 20:1 ratio to Omega-3s, when it should be 4:1). This chronic "fire alarm" state is a driver of autoimmune disease.

Essential Fatty Acids (EFAs): The body is a brilliant chemist, but it has limits. It cannot manufacture Linoleic Acid (Omega-6) or Alpha-Linolenic Acid (Omega-3). We must eat them. Deficiency leads to scaly skin, hair loss, and poor wound healing—a condition rarely seen now but common in patients with fat-malabsorption disorders.

MODULE 3: THE FAB FOUR — SPECIFIC LIPID CLASSES
Functions & Biomedical Deep Dive

Here we enter the specialized machinery. These are the complex lipids that build the body.

A. PHOSPHOLIPIDS (PL): The Gatekeepers

The Function: Phospholipids are "amphipathic," meaning they have a split personality. They have a water-loving (hydrophilic) head and a fat-loving (hydrophobic) tail. When you throw them into water, they spontaneously arrange themselves into a bilayer—heads out, tails in.

The "Fluid Mosaic": They create the matrix of the cell membrane. But they aren't static. They flip, rotate, and move, allowing the cell to change shape (like a white blood cell squeezing through a capillary).

Biomedical Importance:

Lung Surfactant: A specific phospholipid (Dipalmitoylphosphatidylcholine) lines the lungs of newborns. Without it, the air sacs collapse due to surface tension. This is why premature babies often struggle to breathe (Respiratory Distress Syndrome).

Liposomes in Medicine (2026 Update): Remember the COVID-19 mRNA vaccines? They worked because of Lipid Nanoparticles (LNPs)—synthetic cousins of phospholipids. In 2026, we use refined PL spheres to deliver chemotherapy directly inside cancer cells, sparing healthy tissue.

B. LIPOPROTEINS (LP): The Cargo Fleet

The Function: Oil and water don't mix. So, how does the body move fat (oil) through blood (water)? It builds submarines. Lipoproteins are spherical complexes with a hydrophobic core (carrying cholesterol and triglycerides) and a hydrophilic shell (proteins and phospholipids).

The Fleet (by density):

Chylomicrons: The super-tankers. They carry dietary fat from the gut to the body.

VLDL (Very Low Density): The delivery trucks sent from the liver.

LDL (Low Density): The "delivery boys." They drop cholesterol off at cells. (If there are too many, they dump it in the arteries—hence "Bad Cholesterol").

HDL (High Density): The "garbage trucks." They pick up excess cholesterol and take it back to the liver for disposal (Reverse Cholesterol Transport—"Good Cholesterol").

Biomedical Importance (The 2026 View): We have moved beyond just measuring LDL-C.

Lp(a) Screening: In 2026, measuring Lipoprotein(a)—a genetic variant of LDL that is essentially "sticky" and highly clotting-prone—is standard care. It's a silent killer that diet doesn't fix, only genetics dictates.

Proteomics: We now analyze the proteins on the surface of these particles. An HDL particle carrying inflammatory proteins is no longer "good"; it's dysfunctional. This is the era of "Dysfunctional HDL" diagnosis.

C. GLYCOLIPIDS (GL): The Identity Cards

The Function: Glycolipids are lipids with a sugar chain attached. They sit on the outer surface of the cell like antennas or flags.

Cell Recognition: They tell the immune system, "I am part of the body, do not shoot."

Blood Types: The ABO blood group system is actually based on glycolipids on your red blood cells. Type A has one sugar pattern, Type B another.

Biomedical Importance:

Cancer & Immunity: Cancer cells often mutate their glycolipids (shedding their ID cards) to hide from the immune system. New "Glyco-immune" checkpoints drugs in 2026 target these sugar coats to strip the camouflage off tumors.

Cholera Toxin: Bacteria like Vibrio cholerae exploit our glycolipids (specifically GM1 gangliosides) to latch onto gut cells and cause disease.

D. SPHINGOLIPIDS: The Biostats of Life & Death

The Function: Once thought to be just structural (like insulation on nerve fibers—Myelin), we now know they are the Master Regulators.

The Sphingolipid Rheostat: This is a biological see-saw.

Ceramide: The signal for "Stress" and "Death" (Apoptosis).

Sphingosine-1-Phosphate (S1P): The signal for "Survival" and "Proliferation."

The cell constantly balances these two. If the scale tips toward Ceramide, the cell commits suicide. If it tips to S1P, the cell grows (and sometimes becomes cancerous).

Biomedical Importance:

Multiple Sclerosis (MS): This is the classic disease of Sphingolipids. The immune system attacks the sphingomyelin sheath protecting neurons, leading to short-circuits in the nervous system.

Insulin Resistance: In 2026, we understand that in Type 2 Diabetes, it is the accumulation of Ceramide in muscle cells that actually blocks the insulin signal. We are developing drugs that inhibit ceramide synthesis to treat diabetes.

COURSE CONCLUSION: THE LIPID CODE

As we conclude this overview, I want you to look at your hand. Under the skin, billions of cells are functioning. Their membranes are fluid because of unsaturated fatty acids. They are talking to each other using sphingolipids. They are powered by triglycerides. And they are protected by glycolipids.

We have entered the age of Lipidomics. The future of medicine in 2026 and beyond lies in mapping these pathways. We are no longer just treating "high cholesterol"; we are tweaking the sphingolipid rheostat to stop cancer, we are optimizing phospholipid ratios to cure dementia, and we are using lipid nanoparticles to rewrite genetic errors.

Lipids are not just the grease of the biological world; they are the gears, the chips, and the software.

PROTEIN CHEMISTRY

Introduction: The Molecular Architecture of Life

Biochemistry is often called the language of life. It is the discipline that allows us to read the stories written in our blood and tissues. As we settle into 2026, our understanding of this language has shifted dramatically. We no longer view the body as a static machine. We see it as a dynamic, fluctuating ecosystem.

Two critical components of this ecosystem are plasma proteins and amino acids. Think of amino acids as the alphabet. They are the fundamental letters. When arranged in specific orders, they form words and sentences. These sentences are proteins.

When these proteins circulate in our blood, they become plasma proteins. They are the messengers, the defenders, and the builders.

In this deep dive, we will explore these molecules. We will look at them not just as chemical structures, but as active participants in the drama of human health. We will integrate classic knowledge with the breakthroughs of the last few years, including the Nobel-winning AI advances of 2024 and the "deep plasma" profiling that defines clinical science today.

Part 1: Plasma Proteins

1. Defining Plasma Proteins

Blood is a tissue. It is liquid, but it is a tissue nonetheless. If you spin a tube of blood in a centrifuge, the cells sink to the bottom. The liquid that remains on top is straw-colored. This is plasma.

Plasma is mostly water (about 90-92%). But the magic lies in the remaining solute. The most abundant organic solutes in this water are plasma proteins.

By definition, plasma proteins are the diverse group of proteins dissolved in the blood plasma. In a healthy adult, they exist in a concentration of about 6 to 8 grams per deciliter (g/dL). They are not just floating debris. They are the working class of the circulatory system.

Most of these proteins are synthesized in the liver. The liver is the factory. It churns out albumin, fibrinogen, and most globulins. The exceptions are the immunoglobulins (antibodies). These are made by plasma cells (B-lymphocytes) in our lymph nodes and spleen.

The Dynamic Proteome In the past, we thought of plasma proteins as a stable list. Today, in 2026, we view the "plasma proteome" as a shifting sea. Recent studies from 2025 have shown that plasma protein levels "undulate" or move in waves as we age. We now know there are specific crests of protein changes at ages 44, 51, and 63. These proteins define our "metabolic age," which might be very different from the birthday on our driver's license.

2. Classification of Plasma Proteins

We can classify these proteins in two ways. There is the classic method (separation by chemical physics) and the modern method (separation by function).

A. The Classical Classification (Electrophoresis) If we apply an electric current to plasma, the proteins move. They separate based on their charge and size. This gives us five distinct bands.

Albumin: This is the fastest-moving band. It is also the largest. Albumin makes up about 60% of the total protein.

α1-Globulins: The first distinct group after albumin.

α2-Globulins: A slightly slower group.

β-Globulins: The middle group.

γ-Globulins: The slowest group. These are the antibodies.

B. The Functional Classification (The Modern View) In clinical biochemistry, it is often more useful to group them by what they do.

Transport Proteins: These are the taxis of the blood.

Albumin carries fatty acids, calcium, and drugs.

Transferrin carries iron.

Ceruloplasmin carries copper.

Apolipoproteins carry lipids (cholesterol).

Defensive Proteins: These are the soldiers.

Immunoglobulins (IgG, IgM, IgA, etc.) neutralize viruses and bacteria.

Complement proteins circulate in an inactive state but can explode into a "cascade" to punch holes in bacterial walls.

Clotting Proteins: These are the emergency repair crews.

Fibrinogen is the main structural material of a blood clot.

Prothrombin and other clotting factors act as the triggers.

Regulatory Proteins:

This includes hormones (like insulin) and enzymes. Though present in small amounts, their power is immense.

3. Detailed Properties and Functions

Let's zoom in on the major players.

Albumin: The Sponge and the Taxi Albumin is small but mighty. It is a single polypeptide chain. Because it is so abundant and small, it exerts a huge osmotic pressure.

Think of a sponge. Albumin "holds" water in the blood vessels. If albumin levels drop (like in liver failure or starvation), water leaks out of the blood and into the tissues. This causes swelling, or edema. This is the Colloid Osmotic Pressure (COP). Albumin provides about 80% of this pressure.

It is also "sticky." It binds to almost everything. When you take aspirin or penicillin, albumin grabs it and ferries it around the body. This prevents the drug from being excreted too quickly.

The Globulins: Diversity in Action

a1-Antitrypsin: This protein protects our lungs. It neutralizes enzymes that would otherwise digest our own lung tissue. A deficiency here leads to emphysema.

Haptoglobin (α2): This molecule hunts for free hemoglobin. If a red blood cell bursts, hemoglobin is toxic to the kidneys. Haptoglobin binds it instantly to save the kidneys.

C-Reactive Protein (CRP): This is a "fire alarm." Its levels skyrocket when there is inflammation anywhere in the body. In 2026, we now use "high-sensitivity CRP" alongside newer markers to predict heart attacks years in advance.

Fibrinogen: The Net Fibrinogen is a soluble protein. It floats freely. But when the clotting signal is given (by thrombin), it undergoes a radical change. It turns into fibrin. Fibrin is insoluble. It forms a mesh, like a spider web, that traps blood cells to plug a leak.

Part 2: Amino Acids

1. The Alphabet of Biochemistry

If proteins are the house, amino acids are the bricks. But they are smart bricks.

An amino acid is a small organic molecule with a split personality. It has two chemically opposing groups attached to the same central carbon atom (the α-carbon).

A Carboxyl group (−COOH): This is acidic. It wants to donate a proton.

An Amino group (−NH2): This is basic. It wants to accept a proton.

A Hydrogen atom.

A Side chain (R-group): This is the "ID card" of the amino acid. It makes each one unique.

The Zwitterion Nature Because they have both an acid and a base, amino acids rarely exist in the neutral form shown in textbooks. In the watery environment of our cells (pH 7.4), the proton moves from the acid side to the base side.
R−CH(NH2)−COOH⇌R−CH(NH3+)−COO−

This dipolar ion is called a Zwitterion (from the German for "hybrid"). This charge separation is what makes amino acids soluble in water and high-melting. They act like salts.
2. Classification of Amino Acids

There are over 300 amino acids in nature, but our DNA only codes for 20 "standard" ones. We classify them based on the personality of their side chain (R-group).

A. Non-polar (Hydrophobic) These hate water. They act like oil. When a protein folds, these amino acids bury themselves deep inside the structure to hide from the blood.

Examples: Glycine, Alanine, Valine, Leucine, Phenylalanine.

Note: Proline is unique; its side chain loops back to connect to its own backbone, making it rigid.

B. Polar but Uncharged These like water but carry no net charge. They form hydrogen bonds.

Examples: Serine, Threonine, Tyrosine, Cysteine, Glutamine.

Special Mention: Cysteine contains sulfur. Two cysteines can bond to form a "disulfide bridge," which staples proteins together.

C. Acidic (Negatively Charged) These donate protons.

Examples: Aspartic acid, Glutamic acid.

D. Basic (Positively Charged) These accept protons.

Examples: Lysine, Arginine, Histidine.

New Discoveries (2024-2026 Context): While we have known the "Standard 20" for decades, recent research has expanded our view. We now pay close attention to Selenocysteine (the 21st amino acid) and Pyrrolysine. Furthermore, AI tools like AlphaFold 3 (updated in 2025) have allowed us to simulate how "non-standard" amino acids could be used to build synthetic proteins for medicine, creating structures nature never imagined.

3. Properties of Amino Acids

Physical Properties

Solubility: Most are soluble in water but insoluble in organic solvents (like benzene).

Melting Point: They have very high melting points (often above 200°C) because the crystal lattice is held together by strong ionic forces between the zwitterions.

Optical Activity: All amino acids (except Glycine) act like tiny mirrors. They are "chiral." They have a left-handed version (L-isomer) and a right-handed version (D-isomer).

Crucial Fact: Life on Earth is "left-handed." Our proteins are made almost exclusively of L-amino acids. D-amino acids are found mostly in bacterial walls and some antibiotics.

Chemical Properties & Reactions Amino acids are chemically hyper-active. They can react at the acid end, the amino end, or the side chain.

A. Reactions of the Carboxyl Group (−COOH)

Decarboxylation: If you remove the CO2, you get an amine.

Example: Histidine loses CO2 to become Histamine. Histamine is the chemical that causes itching and swelling during allergies.

Amide Formation: The acid can react with ammonia to form an amide.

B. Reactions of the Amino Group (−NH2)

Deamination: The removal of the amino group. This is essential for energy production. The nitrogen is removed (eventually becoming urea) and the carbon skeleton is burned for fuel.

Ninhydrin Test: This is the classic crime-scene reaction. When reacted with Ninhydrin, amino acids turn deep purple (Ruhemann's purple). This detects fingerprints (which contain sweat and amino acids).

C. The Peptide Bond (The Most Important Reaction) This is how life is built. The carboxyl group of one amino acid reacts with the amino group of another. They release a water molecule (H2O) and form a bond.
AminoAcid1+AminoAcid2→Dipeptide+H2O

This bond (−CO−NH−) is rigid and flat. It provides the stability for protein chains.

D. Reactions of the R-Group (Specifics)

Xanthoproteic Reaction: Concentrated nitric acid turns aromatic amino acids (like Tyrosine/Tryptophan) yellow. This is why your skin turns yellow if you accidentally spill nitric acid on it—you are nitrating the proteins in your skin.

Sakaguchi Reaction: Specific for Arginine (turns red).

Sulfur Test: Specific for Cysteine/Methionine (forms black lead sulfide).

E. Advanced Radical Chemistry (2025 Breakthrough) For a long time, we thought stable "radicals" (highly reactive molecules with unpaired electrons) in proteins were limited mostly to Glycine. However, 2025 research has uncovered a new class of enzymes that generate stable radicals on Alanine, Serine, and Threonine. This changes our understanding of enzymatic power. It suggests that amino acids are capable of far more exotic chemistry than we previously taught.

Conclusion: The Integrated View

As we conclude this analysis, the connection between amino acids and plasma proteins becomes clear. Amino acids are the raw materials. Through the miracle of peptide bonding and folding—predicted now with near-perfect accuracy by AI—they become the functional plasma proteins.

The liver synthesizes these proteins, constantly replacing the old with the new. This turnover is vital. It allows the blood to adapt to stress, infection, and age.

From the simple glycine molecule to the massive immunoglobulin complex, this system is a masterpiece of chemical engineering. In 2026, with the aid of "deep plasma" proteomics, we are no longer just observing these molecules. We are beginning to use them to predict the future of a patient's health.

The study of Biochemistry is the study of these connections. It is the realization that a single change in an amino acid sequence can alter a plasma protein, which can, in turn, change the fate of a human life.

1. Introduction: The Machines of Life

Proteins are not just nutrients on a food label. They are the molecular machines that run every millisecond of biological time. If DNA is the blueprint of life, proteins are the construction workers, the bricks, the engines, and the demolition crews.

For decades, we believed a protein's function was strictly defined by its 3D shape—a rigid "lock and key." But as we stand here in 2026, looking back at the breakthrough Nobel Prize of 2024 awarded to Baker, Hassabis, and Jumper for AlphaFold and computational design, we know the truth is more dynamic. We can now predict protein structures with near-perfect accuracy using AI. We can even design proteins that never existed in nature to cure diseases.

This coursework explores proteins from their atomic roots to their vital role in human blood plasma. We will look at the "classic" science and the "new" biology of disordered regions and liquid droplets.

2. The Structure of Proteins: From Beads to Blueprints

Proteins are polymers. This means they are long chains made of smaller, repeating units. Imagine a pearl necklace. The necklace is the protein; the pearls are amino acids.

2.1 The Building Blocks: Amino Acids

There are 20 standard amino acids found in the human body. Each one has a "personality" based on its chemical side chain:

Hydrophobic (Water-fearing): These hide inside the protein to escape water.

Hydrophilic (Water-loving): These stay on the outside to interact with blood and cytoplasm.

Charged (Positive or Negative): These act like magnets, attracting or repelling other molecules.

2.2 The Four Levels of Architecture

Biochemists divide protein structure into four levels. You must understand this hierarchy to understand disease.

1. Primary Structure (The Sequence) This is the specific order of amino acids in the chain. It is determined directly by your genes.

Example: If you change just one amino acid in the chain of Hemoglobin (glutamic acid to valine), the protein collapses. This causes Sickle Cell Anemia. A single "typo" in the sequence can be fatal.

2. Secondary Structure (The Fold) The chain does not stay straight. It twists and folds due to hydrogen bonds.

Alpha-helix: A spiral shape, like a telephone cord (common in wool/keratin).

Beta-sheet: A flat, pleated shape, like a folded paper fan (common in silk).

3. Tertiary Structure (The 3D Shape) This is the final global shape of the protein. The helices and sheets fold over each other. This folding is driven by the "hydrophobic effect"—oily parts tucking inside to avoid water.

Analogy: Think of a piece of origami. The paper (primary) is folded (secondary) into a crane (tertiary).

4. Quaternary Structure (The Team) Some proteins are too big to be just one chain. They are made of multiple chains clumping together.

Example: Hemoglobin is a team of four subunits. If they don't stick together correctly, they cannot carry oxygen efficiently.

2.3 The "New" Biology: Intrinsically Disordered Proteins (IDPs)

Advanced Concept: For a long time, textbooks said a protein must have a fixed shape to work. We now know this is wrong. About 30% of your proteins are Intrinsically Disordered Proteins (IDPs). They are shape-shifters. They have no fixed structure. They flop around like spaghetti until they meet a partner.

Why is this important? This flexibility allows them to bind to many different partners, not just one. This is crucial for signaling and cancer regulation.

3. The Functional Spectrum

Proteins do almost everything. We can categorize their jobs into a few key sectors.

3.1 Catalysis (Enzymes)

Enzymes are catalysts. They speed up reactions that would otherwise take millions of years.

Example: Amylase in your saliva turns bread starch into sugar instantly. Without enzymes, digestion is impossible.

3.2 Structure and Support

Some proteins are essentially biological cement or steel beams.

Collagen: The most abundant protein in your body. It holds your skin and bones together.

Keratin: The waterproof armor that makes up your hair, nails, and skin surface.

3.3 Transport and Storage

Proteins act as taxis and warehouses.

Hemoglobin: Taxis oxygen from lungs to tissues.

Ferritin: Stores iron in the liver so it doesn't become toxic.

3.4 Motion

Muscle contraction is purely protein-based.

Actin and Myosin: These two proteins slide past each other to shorten muscle fibers. Every time you blink or walk, these proteins are ratcheting together.

3.5 The "New" Function: Biomolecular Condensates

2026 Update: We recently discovered that proteins can form "liquid droplets" inside the cell, a process called Liquid-Liquid Phase Separation (LLPS). Imagine oil droplets in water. Proteins can do this to create "factories" inside the cell without needing a membrane wall. This concentrates reactions in one spot.

Biomedical link: In diseases like ALS (Lou Gehrig's Disease), these liquid droplets harden into solid glass-like clumps, killing the neuron.

4. Biomedical Importance of Proteins

Why do medical students study proteins? Because nearly every drug targets a protein, and nearly every disease involves a broken one.

4.1 Proteins as Drug Targets

Most drugs work by sticking to a protein and turning it off or on.

Example: Aspirin works by blocking a protein enzyme (Cyclooxygenase) that signals pain.

Modern Tech: PROTACs (Proteolysis Targeting Chimeras) are a new class of drugs that don't just block a "bad" protein—they tag it for destruction by the cell's own waste disposal system.

4.2 Nutritional Deficiency

If you don't eat enough protein, the body cannibalizes its own muscles.

Kwashiorkor: A disease of severe protein deficiency. The belly swells because there is not enough albumin in the blood to hold water in the vessels (we will discuss this in the Plasma section).

4.3 Protein Misfolding Diseases

If a protein folds wrong, it can become toxic.

Alzheimer's Disease: Caused by "Amyloid beta" and "Tau" proteins clumping up in the brain.

Prion Diseases (Mad Cow): A scary scenario where a misfolded protein infects other healthy proteins, forcing them to misfold too.

5. Biomedical Importance of Simple Proteins (Plasma Proteins)

We now focus on a specific group: the proteins floating in your blood. These are often called "Simple Proteins" because they yield only amino acids upon hydrolysis (breakdown), unlike complex proteins which might have metals or sugars attached.

Blood plasma is a busy highway. It contains over 3000 different proteins, but we focus on the "Big Three": Albumin, Globulins, and Fibrinogen.

5.1 Albumin: The Universal Carrier

Albumin is the most abundant protein in plasma (about 55-60%). It is made by the liver.

Function 1: Osmotic Pressure. Albumin acts like a sponge. It keeps water inside your blood vessels. If albumin levels drop, water leaks out into the tissues.

Clinical Consequence: Edema (swelling). This is why liver failure patients often have swollen abdomens (ascites)—their liver stopped making albumin.

Function 2: The Taxi. Many drugs and hormones are not water-soluble. They cannot float in blood alone. Albumin grabs them and carries them.

Example: Calcium, fatty acids, and many antibiotics ride on albumin.

5.2 Globulins: The Defenders

These are heavier than albumin. They are divided into alpha, beta, and gamma globulins.

Alpha & Beta Globulins: mostly transport vehicles (e.g., Transferrin carries iron).

Gamma Globulins (Immunoglobulins): These are Antibodies. They are the soldiers of the immune system. They recognize and neutralize viruses and bacteria.

Clinical Consequence: If you lack gamma globulins, you have "agammaglobulinemia" and are prone to severe, recurrent infections.

5.3 Fibrinogen: The Glue

This is a large protein involved in clotting. When you cut yourself, an enzyme clips Fibrinogen, turning it into Fibrin. Fibrin forms a mesh net that catches blood cells to plug the hole.

Clinical Consequence: Hemophiliacs or people with liver disease may lack clotting factors, leading to uncontrolled bleeding.

5.4 2026 Diagnostic Breakthroughs: Plasma Biomarkers

The analysis of plasma proteins is revolutionizing medicine right now.

The p-tau217 Revolution: In the past, diagnosing Alzheimer's required painful spinal taps or expensive brain scans. Recent 2024-2025 studies confirmed that a simple blood test measuring a plasma protein called p-tau217 can detect Alzheimer's pathology with over 90% accuracy. This is a game-changer for early detection.

Proteomics Panels: Instead of checking one protein, doctors can now scan thousands of plasma proteins at once (using tools like the UK Biobank dataset) to predict heart attacks or cancer years before symptoms appear.

6. Conclusion

Proteins are the workforce of life. From the rigid keratin in your fingernails to the shapeless, dancing IDPs in your neurons, they dictate health and disease.

In 2026, we have moved beyond just looking at protein structures. We are now predicting them with AI and manipulating them with new drugs. The study of plasma proteins has shifted from simple liver function tests to advanced "liquid biopsies" that can detect dementia from a finger-prick of blood.

Understanding proteins is not just biochemistry; it is the key to the future of personalized medicine.

ENZYMES

Introduction: The Spark of Life

Imagine a city without traffic lights, construction crews, or waste management systems. It would be chaos. Nothing would move. Nothing would get built. That is a cell without enzymes.

In this course module, we are going to explore the biological machines that make life possible. We are not just going to memorize definitions. We are going to look under the hood of the most efficient engines in the universe.

You have asked for a complete account. We will cover the fundamentals, the rigid classification systems used globally, and the cutting-edge science emerging right now in 2026.

Part 1: Defining Enzymes (The Molecular Choreographers)

What is an Enzyme?

At its simplest level, an enzyme is a biological catalyst. But that definition is too dry. Think of an enzyme as a molecular matchmaker.

Chemical reactions want to happen, but they are often shy. They need a huge amount of energy to get started. This energy barrier is called "activation energy." Without help, a sugar molecule might sit on your table for years without breaking down.

Enzymes change the game. They grab the molecules (substrates), hold them in the perfect position, and lower that energy barrier. They make the impossible, possible. And they make the slow, instant.

The Composition: More Than Just Protein

Most enzymes are proteins. They are long chains of amino acids folded into complex 3D shapes. But they are not always alone.

Apoenzyme: This is the protein part. It is like the engine block of a car.

Cofactor: This is the key. Some enzymes need a non-protein helper to work. If it is an organic molecule (like Vitamin B), we call it a Coenzyme. If it is a metal ion (like Iron or Magnesium), it is just a cofactor.

Holoenzyme: When the protein and the helper come together, they form the complete, active "holoenzyme."

Example: Hemoglobin needs iron to carry oxygen. Without the iron, the protein is useless.

The Active Site: Where Magic Happens

Enzymes are huge, but the work happens in a tiny pocket called the active site. This is a specific groove on the surface of the protein.

For a long time, scientists taught the "Lock and Key" model. They thought the substrate fit into the enzyme perfectly, like a key in a lock. We now know this is too simple.

In 2026, we focus on the "Induced Fit" model. Imagine a handshake. As your hand meets another, both hands change shape slightly to get a firm grip. Enzymes do the same. As the substrate enters, the enzyme clamps down around it. This shape-shifting puts stress on the chemical bonds, snapping them or forging new ones.

Part 2: The Classification of Enzymes (The EC System)

Biology loves order. To keep track of the thousands of enzymes we have discovered, we use a standard system called the Enzyme Commission (EC) number.

Until recently, textbooks listed six classes. But science evolves. As of the latest IUBMB standards (fully integrated into 2026 coursework), we now recognize seven distinct classes of enzymes.

Here is your deep dive into the seven pillars of enzymology.

Class 1: Oxidoreductases (The Energy Traders)

These are the power plants of the cell. They handle electron transfer. Life is essentially a flow of electrons, and these enzymes direct that flow. They take electrons (and often hydrogen) from one molecule and give them to another.

What they do: Oxidation (losing electrons) and Reduction (gaining electrons).

The Reaction: Areduced+Boxidized→Aoxidized +Breduced

Real-World Example: Alcohol Dehydrogenase. When you drink a glass of wine, this enzyme in your liver strips hydrogen from the ethanol to break it down. It is the reason you can metabolize alcohol.

Class 2: Transferases (The Movers)

These enzymes are the delivery trucks. They pick up a functional group—like a phosphate, a methyl group, or a sugar—from one molecule and move it to another.

What they do: Group transfer.

The Reaction: $A-X+B \rightarrow A+B-X$

Real-World Example: Hexokinase. This is the first step of glycolysis (sugar burning). It grabs a phosphate group from ATP (energy currency) and attaches it to glucose. This "tags" the glucose so the cell can use it.

Class 3: Hydrolases (The Breakers)

These are the demolition crew. They break chemical bonds by adding water. This is the main type of enzyme used in your digestive system to break down food.

What they do: Hydrolysis (breaking with water).

The Reaction: $A-B+H2O \rightarrow A-H+B-OH$

Real-World Example: Lactase. This enzyme breaks down lactose (milk sugar). If you don't have enough Lactase, the lactose stays intact and causes gas and bloating—that is lactose intolerance.

Class 4: Lyases (The Cutters)

These are like surgical scissors. They break bonds without using water and without moving electrons. They usually leave behind a double bond, or they add a group to a double bond.

What they do: Non-hydrolytic cleavage.

The Reaction: $A-B \rightarrow A=B+X$

Real-World Example: Pyruvate Decarboxylase. It removes a carbon atom from pyruvate, releasing it as CO_2. This is the enzyme in yeast that makes bread dough rise (the bubbles are CO_2).

Class 5: Isomerases (The Shifters)

These are the magicians. They don't add anything or take anything away. They simply rearrange the atoms inside a molecule to change its shape.

What they do: Intramolecular rearrangement.

The Reaction: $A \rightarrow iso-A$

Real-World Example: Phosphoglucoisomerase. In glycolysis, this enzyme turns Glucose-6-phosphate into Fructose-6-phosphate. Same atoms, different shape. It is a necessary shuffle to prepare the molecule for the next step.

Class 6: Ligases (The Builders)

These are the construction workers. They join two large molecules together. But building requires effort. These enzymes almost always need energy, usually in the form of ATP, to bond the molecules.

What they do: Joining of two molecules (Synthesis).

The Reaction: $A+B+ATP \rightarrow A-B+ADP+Pi$

Real-World Example: DNA Ligase. This is the glue of genetics. When DNA is replicated or repaired, DNA Ligase seals the breaks in the backbone, ensuring your genetic code remains intact.

Class 7: Translocases (The Porters)

This is the "new" class that older textbooks might miss, but it is standard in 2026. These enzymes are unique because their job isn't just to change a molecule, but to move it across a membrane.

What they do: Movement of ions or molecules across membranes.

The Context: Previously, we thought of these just as "pumps." But because they use ATP hydrolysis (a chemical reaction) to drive movement, they are classified as enzymes.

Real-World Example: ATP Synthase. This sits in your mitochondria. It moves protons across a membrane to generate ATP. It is literally the motor that powers your life.

Part 3: The 2026 Frontier (New Information)

You asked for the latest, verifiable information. The field of enzymology has shifted drastically in the last two years. We are no longer just discovering enzymes; we are designing them.

1. AI-Driven De Novo Design (The "CleaveNet" Breakthrough)

As of January 2026, the biggest story in biochemistry is the move from "structure prediction" to "function generation."

In the past, we used tools like AlphaFold to predict what an enzyme looked like. Now, we use Generative AI models to design enzymes from scratch.

The Breakthrough: Just this week (Jan 2026), researchers at MIT released a study on a system called "CleaveNet."

How it works: Instead of looking for a natural enzyme that might work, they used AI to design synthetic peptides and enzymes specifically tailored to detect cancer. These enzymes are designed to be "hyper-active" only in the presence of specific cancer markers.

Why it matters: This isn't just biology; it is engineering. We are writing genetic code to build machines that evolution never created.

2. Synzymes (Synthetic Enzymes)

We are seeing the rise of "Synzymes." These are enzymes designed to catalyze reactions that do not exist in nature.

Example: Nature has no enzyme to form a carbon-silicon bond. But in 2025, scientists engineered variants of Cytochrome c (normally an electron carrier) to force this bond to happen. This opens the door to biologically manufacturing silicon chips or new types of biodegradable plastics.

3. The Plastic Eaters (Polymer Depolymerases)

By 2026, the focus on plastic pollution has led to the optimization of PETase (an enzyme that eats plastic bottles).

The Update: Early versions of this enzyme were slow and melted at high temperatures. Using AI, scientists have now created "Thermo-PETase." This variant is stable at 70°C (158°F), which is crucial because plastic degrades much faster when it is warm and soft. We are now seeing pilot plants where these enzymes digest tons of plastic waste into reusable raw materials.

Conclusion

Enzymes are the laborers of life. They are the reason you can breathe, move, digest food, and read this sentence.

We defined them as biological catalysts that lower activation energy. We classified them into seven distinct families: Oxidoreductases, Transferases, Hydrolases, Lyases, Isomerases, Ligases, and the recently formalized Translocases.

But the most exciting takeaway for your coursework is this: Enzymology is no longer a static science. With the help of Artificial Intelligence, we have stopped waiting for nature to solve our problems. In 2026, we are designing the enzymes we need to cure diseases, clean the ocean, and power the future.

This concludes the module on Enzymes.

Introduction: The Molecular Engines of Life

Imagine a city where millions of tasks must happen every second—traffic directing, waste recycling, construction, and energy production. If these tasks relied on random chance, the city would collapse instantly. In the cellular metropolis, enzymes are the specialized workers that ensure these processes occur not just eventually, but immediately.

Enzymes are biological catalysts. In simple terms, they speed up chemical reactions without being consumed by them. Without enzymes, the digestion of a single meal could take weeks; with them, it takes hours. For decades, we viewed enzymes as rigid "locks" waiting for "keys." However, as we stand here in 2026, our understanding has shifted dramatically. We no longer see them merely as static biological hardware but as dynamic, breathing entities—and thanks to the explosion of Artificial Intelligence (AI) in biochemistry over the last two years, we are no longer just studying them; we are building them from scratch.

This coursework provides a deep dive into the physical structure of enzymes, how they perform their chemical magic, and the mathematical laws—specifically the Michaelis-Menten equation—that govern their speed. We will also explore the groundbreaking discoveries of 2024 and 2025 that have rewritten textbooks, including the creation of enzymes for reactions nature never intended.

Part 1: The Architecture of Enzymes

To understand what an enzyme does, we must first look at what it is.

1.1 The Structural Hierarchy

Most enzymes are proteins (though some RNA molecules, called ribozymes, also act as catalysts). Their function is entirely dictated by their three-dimensional shape.

Primary Structure: This is the specific sequence of amino acids linked by peptide bonds. Think of this as the letters in a sentence. If you misspell a word (a mutation), the sentence might lose its meaning.

Secondary Structure: Local folding patterns, such as alpha-helices (coils) and beta-sheets (flat folds), stabilized by hydrogen bonds.

Tertiary Structure: The overall 3D shape of the single protein molecule. This is where the magic happens. Hydrophobic (water-fearing) parts hide inside, while hydrophilic (water-loving) parts face the cellular fluid.

Quaternary Structure: Some enzymes are teams. They consist of multiple protein subunits working together (e.g., Hemoglobin or the massive Pyruvate Dehydrogenase complex).

1.2 The Active Site: The Engine Room

The massive bulk of an enzyme often serves just one purpose: to position a tiny cleft called the active site. This is where the substrate (the molecule being acted upon) binds.

Classically, we were taught the "Lock and Key" model (Emil Fischer, 1894), suggesting the active site acts like a rigid keyhole. However, modern science favors the "Induced Fit" model (Daniel Koshland). Imagine a hand slipping into a glove; the glove changes shape slightly to mold around the hand. Similarly, as a substrate approaches, the enzyme shifts its shape to hug the substrate tighter.

2026 Update: The "Ensemble" View Recent findings from Stanford and time-resolved crystallography in late 2025 have pushed us beyond "Induced Fit." We now understand that enzymes exist in "conformational ensembles." They are not twitching between two states (open and closed) but are vibrating through a landscape of shapes. The substrate merely selects the shape that works best. This "shapeshifting" is crucial. For instance, recent X-ray snapshots of the enzyme N-RAS (a cancer-linked protein) revealed over 57 distinct intermediate shapes during a single reaction cycle. This level of detail was unimaginable just five years ago.

Part 2: Mechanism of Action

How does an enzyme actually make a reaction faster? It all comes down to energy.

2.1 Lowering the Activation Energy

Every chemical reaction requires an initial energy investment to start—like pushing a boulder up a hill before it can roll down the other side. This peak is the Transition State. Enzymes work by lowering the height of this hill. They stabilize the transition state, making it easier for the molecules to reach that tipping point.

Analogy: If you need to break a stick (the reaction), you could bend it until it snaps. An enzyme acts like a vice that holds the stick bent (the transition state), so you barely need to touch it to break it.

2.2 Catalytic Strategies

Enzymes use several chemical tricks to stabilize the transition state:

Acid-Base Catalysis: The enzyme donates or steals protons (H^+) to make the substrate more reactive. Residues like Histidine are famous for this because they can swap protons easily at body pH.

Covalent Catalysis: The enzyme temporarily forms a chemical bond with the substrate. It holds the molecule tight, performs the change, and then releases it.

Metal Ion Catalysis: Many enzymes use metal helpers (cofactors) like Zinc (Zn^{2+}) or Iron (Fe^{2+}). These metals act like electron magnets, stabilizing negative charges that would otherwise be unstable.

Proximity and Orientation: The enzyme grabs two molecules and forces them together in exactly the right alignment. It's the difference between tossing keys at a lock from across the room versus carefully inserting the key.

2.3 The 2026 Breakthrough: "BioHAT" and Radical Chemistry

Historically, we thought nature had a limited "playbook" of reaction types. However, a major 2025 breakthrough by a team at UCLA shattered this assumption. They engineered an enzyme to perform "BioHAT" (Biocatalytic Hydrogen Atom Transfer).

Nature usually moves hydrogens as pairs (hydride transfer). This new artificial enzyme moves single hydrogen atoms (radicals) using an iron center. This mechanism allows the enzyme to process industrial chemicals (alkenes) in water at room temperature—something that previously required toxic metals and high pressure. This proves that enzymes are not limited to "natural" biology; they can be reprogrammed for alien chemistry.

Part 3: Enzyme Kinetics & The Michaelis-Menten Equation

To control enzymes (for drugs or industry), we need to measure their speed. This brings us to the mathematical heart of enzymology: Kinetics.

3.1 The Michaelis-Menten Model

Proposed in 1913 by Leonor Michaelis and Maud Menten, this model describes how reaction rate (v) depends on substrate concentration ([S]).

The basic equation is:
v0=Km+[S]Vmax[S]

Where:

v0: The initial speed of the reaction.

Vmax: The maximum possible speed. This happens when every single enzyme molecule is busy working (saturation).

[S]: The concentration of substrate.

Km (Michaelis Constant): This is the concentration of substrate needed to reach exactly half of Vmax.

Why is Km important? Km tells us about affinity.

Low Km: The enzyme loves the substrate. It works fast even with very little substrate present.

High Km: The enzyme is picky. It needs a lot of substrate to get going.

3.2 The Turnover Number (kcat)

Vmax depends on how much enzyme you have. A more intrinsic measure is kcat, or the turnover number.
kcat=[E]totalVmax

This tells you how many molecules of product one single enzyme molecule can churn out per second. Some enzymes are slow (1 per second); others, like Carbonic Anhydrase, are beasts, converting 600,000 molecules per second!

3.3 Catalytic Efficiency (kcat/Km)

This is the ultimate scorecard for an enzyme. It combines speed (kcat) and grip (Km). An enzyme with high efficiency is "perfect"—it converts substrate almost instantly upon collision.

3.4 Recent Deviations (The 2026 Context)

For over a century, we assumed MM kinetics worked universally. However, 2025 research using single-molecule fluorescence spectroscopy has shown that at very high substrate concentrations, enzymes "break" the MM law.

The variance in turnover times becomes "multiexponential." This means the enzyme isn't just resetting instantly; it gets "tired" or stuck in different shape-states that process substrate at different speeds. This "dynamic disorder" is a hot topic in 2026 because it affects how we model drug metabolism in the liver. New "Modified MM Equations" are now being used in computational pharmacology (PBPK modeling) to predict drug interactions more accurately than the classical equation ever could.

Part 4: Regulation and Inhibition

Enzymes must be switchable. You don't want digestive enzymes active inside the cells that make them (or they'd eat the cell!).

4.1 Inhibition

Drugs are often enzyme inhibitors. They stop a specific reaction to cure a disease.

Competitive Inhibition: The drug looks like the substrate and steals the active site. (Effect: Km increases, Vmax stays same). Example: Ibuprofen blocks pain enzymes.

Non-Competitive Inhibition: The drug attaches to the back of the enzyme, distorting the active site. (Effect: Vmax drops, Km stays same).

Uncompetitive Inhibition: The drug only binds after the substrate is already locked in. This is rare but potent.

4.2 Allosteric Regulation

This is the "dimer switch" of biology. An allosteric enzyme has a secondary site (allosteric site). When a regulator molecule binds there, the active site changes shape.

Cooperativity: In multi-subunit enzymes, if one unit binds a substrate, the others snap open to help. This creates a "sigmoidal" (S-shaped) curve on a graph, rather than the smooth MM hyperbola. This is crucial for metabolic control—it allows enzymes to be super-sensitive to small changes in substrate levels.

Part 5: The Future is Now (2026 Innovations)

The field of Biochemistry has transformed from observation to creation.

5.1 AI-Driven De Novo Design

In 2024 and 2025, tools like AlphaFold 3 and RFdiffusion (from the Baker Lab) allowed us to design proteins that do not exist in nature.

Case Study: SNAr1.3: In early 2025, researchers evolved a completely new enzyme to perform nucleophilic aromatic substitution (SNAr). This reaction creates bonds vital for pharmaceuticals. Nature had no enzyme for this. We built one. It operates in water, replacing dirty industrial solvents.

Amide Bond Synthesis: Another 2025 breakthrough involved using Machine Learning (ML) to map the fitness landscape of amide synthetases (McbA). This allows us to "print" enzymes tailored to build specific new drugs, slashing development time.

5.2 Green Chemistry

The push for sustainability (Net Zero) is driving enzymology. We are replacing heavy metal catalysts (palladium, platinum) with engineered enzymes. These "biocatalysts" work at room temperature and pressure, drastically reducing the carbon footprint of chemical manufacturing.

Conclusion

We have journeyed from the atomic arrangement of amino acids to the mathematical curves of Michaelis-Menten, and finally to the AI-designed frontiers of 2026.

Enzymes are more than just catalysts; they are the nanomachines that bridge the gap between non-living chemistry and living biology. The classical laws of kinetics still hold, but our "2026 eyes" see the nuance—the vibration of the protein structure, the slight deviations in single-molecule behavior, and the limitless potential of artificial enzymes.

As we look forward, the distinction between "natural" biology and "synthetic" chemistry is blurring. We are entering an era where if a chemical reaction is possible, we can build an enzyme to drive it. The student of biochemistry today is not just memorizing pathways, but learning the logic to design the molecular future.

References & Further Reading (2025-2026 Context):

Nature (Jan 2025): "Discovery of SNAr1.3 and Nucleophilic Aromatic Substitution in Water."

Science (Feb 2025): "Ensemble Views of Enzyme Catalysis via Time-Resolved Crystallography."

Journal of Physical Chemistry B (2025): "Deviations from MM Kinetics in Single-Enzyme Turnover."

UCLA Chemistry Reports (Nov 2025): "BioHAT: Radical Hydrogenation Mechanisms in Artificial Enzymes."

Introduction: The Molecular Decision Makers

Welcome to the deep dive into Enzymology. If you were to look at a cell not as a biological blob, but as a bustling city, enzymes would not just be the construction workers; they would be the traffic lights, the foremen, the demolition crews, and the architects all rolled into one. Without them, the chemical reactions that sustain life would happen so slowly that a single heartbeat might take a thousand years.

In this unit, we are moving beyond the high school definition of "biological catalysts." We are going to explore enzymes as dynamic, breathing molecular machines that are sensitive to their environment, rigorously controlled by the cell, and increasingly used by doctors to diagnose illness and cure genetic diseases. We will integrate foundational biochemistry with the cutting-edge reality of 2026, where Artificial Intelligence and nanotechnology are rewriting the rules of what enzymes can do.

Section 1: Factors Affecting Enzyme Activity (The Environment Matters)

Enzymes are protein divas. They are incredibly powerful, capable of accelerating reactions by a factor of millions, but they are also high-maintenance. They demand specific conditions to perform their "molecular dance." If the lights are too bright (wrong pH) or the room is too hot (high temperature), they simply refuse to work.

1. Temperature: The Goldilocks Zone

You might have heard that "heat increases reaction rates." This is true in a test tube of simple chemicals because heat is just kinetic energy—it makes molecules bang into each other harder and faster. But enzymes are delicate 3D puzzles held together by weak bonds.

The Rise: As you warm up an enzymatic reaction, the rate climbs. The substrate (the molecule the enzyme acts on) collides with the enzyme's active site more frequently.

The Fall: Suddenly, you hit a tipping point—usually around 40°C for human enzymes. The thermal energy becomes too violent for the weak hydrogen bonds holding the enzyme's shape. The protein unravels, or denatures. Imagine melting a plastic key; it might still look like plastic, but it will never open the lock again.

2026 Perspective: Today, we are no longer limited by nature's fragility. In 2026, we are seeing the rise of "Nanozymes"—artificial nanomaterials that mimic enzyme active sites but are made of robust metals or carbon. Unlike fragile proteins, these can withstand boiling temperatures, making them revolutionary for industrial manufacturing and cancer treatments where the environment is harsh.

2. pH: The Electrical Landscape

Enzymes work via electric charges. The active site often uses positive or negative residues to pull and push on the substrate's electrons.

The Mechanism: If you change the pH, you change the ionization state of these residues. An aspartate residue that needs to be negatively charged might grab a proton in acidic conditions and become neutral. Suddenly, the magnetic attraction is gone.

Context is King: Pepsin in your stomach loves acid (pH 2), while Trypsin in your intestine prefers a slightly basic environment (pH 8). If you swapped them, they would both stop working immediately.

3. Substrate Concentration: The Traffic Jam

Imagine a toll booth (the enzyme) and cars (the substrate).

First Order Kinetics: At first, adding more cars increases the number of people getting through.

Zero Order Kinetics (Saturation): Eventually, the toll booth operator is working as fast as physically possible. Adding more cars doesn't speed up the process; it just creates a line. This maximum speed is called Vmax.

The Clinical Reality: In the human body, we rarely operate at Vmax. We usually operate at a speed sensitive to changes in substrate, allowing the enzyme to speed up or slow down as needed.

Section 2: The Control Room (Regulation of Enzyme Activity)

If enzymes worked at full speed 100% of the time, we would burn through our fuel reserves in minutes and overheat. The cell needs braking systems and accelerators.

1. Allosteric Regulation: The Dimmer Switch

This is the most elegant form of control. "Allosteric" means "other shape."

How it works: An allosteric enzyme has a front door (active site) and a back door (allosteric site). A regulator molecule binds to the back door, causing a ripple effect through the protein structure that either clamps the front door shut (inhibition) or pries it open (activation).

2026 Breakthrough: For decades, "undruggable" proteins like the GTPases (involved in cancer) defied treatment because their active sites were too smooth. In late 2025 and early 2026, we saw the explosion of AI-driven Allosteric Drug Design. Models like AlloPED and CleaveNet are now predicting hidden "pockets" on these enzymes that don't look like binding sites to a human eye but are perfect targets for drugs that "freeze" the enzyme in an off position. This is changing how we treat pancreatic and lung cancers.

2. Covalent Modification: The On/Off Switch

While allosteric control is temporary (like holding a button down), covalent modification is like flipping a switch.

Phosphorylation: The most common method. An enzyme called a kinase adds a heavy phosphate group to a target enzyme. This negative charge forces the protein to change shape. It's the cellular equivalent of slapping a "Do Not Disturb" or "Open for Business" sign on the enzyme.

Zymogens: Some enzymes are too dangerous to be built "active." Proteases (protein-eaters) in the pancreas would digest the pancreas itself if they were active immediately. Instead, they are built as zymogens—inactive precursors with a safety lock. Only when they reach the intestine is the "safety" cut off (proteolytic cleavage), activating the weapon.

3. Feedback Inhibition: The Thermostat

In a factory line, if you have too much final product, you tell the first person in the line to stop working. In biochemistry, the final product of a pathway often floats back and binds to the first enzyme in the chain, shutting it down. This prevents waste.

Section 3: Clinical Significance of Enzymes (The Medical Frontier)

In 2026, enzymes are the cornerstone of modern medicine, serving two roles: Biomarkers (clues to what is wrong) and Therapeutics (the cure itself).

A. Enzymes as Diagnostics (The Leaking Cell Theory)

When cells die or get damaged, their internal enzymes spill into the blood. By measuring which enzymes are high, we can pinpoint exactly which organ is screaming for help.

Heart Attacks (Myocardial Infarction):

The Old Way: We used to look for CK-MB (Creatine Kinase).

The Standard: We now look for Cardiac Troponins (proteins regulated by enzymes).

The 2026 Future: We are moving toward Multi-omics. Instead of just one enzyme, we use AI to analyze patterns of dozens of enzymes simultaneously. This allows us to predict a heart attack before the damage is irreversible, detecting "molecular stress" rather than just cell death.

Liver Function:

ALT & AST: These enzymes handle amino acids in the liver. If your liver is inflamed (hepatitis, alcohol abuse), these leak out.

The Ratio: The ratio of AST to ALT is a subtle code. An AST:ALT ratio greater than 2:1 is the classic "signature" of alcoholic liver disease.

The Cancer Revolution (Protease Activity Sensors):

Here is where the "New Information" gets exciting. Cancer cells are invasive; they use enzymes called Matrix Metalloproteinases (MMPs) to chew through tissue so they can spread.

2026 Technology: We now have "synthetic biomarkers." Scientists at MIT and Microsoft have designed nanoparticles coated in specific peptides. You inhale or swallow them. If—and only if—you have a tumor releasing those specific MMPs, the nanoparticles get "cut." The cut pieces are then urinated out. A simple urine test on a paper strip can now detect lung or colon cancer months before a CT scan would see a tumor. This is the CleaveNet system, and it represents a shift from imaging cancer to sensing its enzymatic activity.

B. Enzymes as Drugs (Therapeutics)

We don't just measure enzymes; we inject them.

Enzyme Replacement Therapy (ERT):

For children born with genetic errors (like Gaucher's or Pompe disease) where a single lysosomal enzyme is missing, waste builds up in their cells like trash in a city without sanitation.

We now manufacture these enzymes in bioreactors and inject them. In 2025, the FDA approved new brain-penetrating enzymes for Alpha-Mannosidosis, crossing the blood-brain barrier that previously stopped these drugs from working on neurological symptoms.

CRISPR as an Enzymatic Drug:

We often call CRISPR "gene editing," but at its core, Cas9 is an endonuclease—an enzyme that cuts DNA.

The 2026 Update: We are seeing the second generation of these enzymatic drugs. CTX310, a liver-editing CRISPR therapy, uses this enzyme to permanently disable the ANGPTL3 gene, lowering cholesterol by 80% with a single dose. We are effectively using an enzyme to perform "molecular surgery" on the genome.

Conclusion: The Engines of Adaptation

In summary, enzymes are the bridge between the inert chemistry of the universe and the dynamic complexity of life. Their activity is not static; it is a constantly shifting equilibrium affected by heat, pH, and strict regulatory controls like allostery and phosphorylation.

Clinically, we have moved from simply observing enzymes (diagnosing liver failure or heart attacks) to mastering them. Whether it is designing artificial nanozymes to fight cancer or using CRISPR endonucleases to cure genetic heart disease, the field of enzymology in 2026 is no longer just about understanding how life works—it is about rewriting the code to make life work better.

NUCLEOPROTEINS

Introduction: The Language of Life

Biology, at its most fundamental level, is an information science. Before we can understand the complex physiology of an organism, we must understand the code in which it is written. In this module, we will deconstruct the molecular alphabet (Nucleotides) and the grammar rules that govern how this alphabet creates meaning (The Central Dogma).

Note for 2026 Students: We are no longer looking at these structures as static entities. The research landscape of 2024-2025 has revolutionized our understanding. We now know the "Central Dogma" is not a rigid one-way street but a complex, regulated highway with "off-ramps," "u-turns," and "traffic control" mediated by epitranscriptomics and synthetic base pairs.

Part I: Nucleotides – The Alphabet of Existence

1. Definition and Fundamental Structure

A nucleotide is the fundamental monomeric unit of nucleic acids (DNA and RNA). It is the molecular "brick" that builds the genome. However, unlike a simple clay brick, a nucleotide is a tripartite machine capable of carrying energy, signaling messages, and acting as a cofactor for enzymes.

Every nucleotide consists of three distinct chemical components covalently linked together:

A Pentose Sugar: A five-carbon sugar ring. In RNA (Ribonucleic Acid), this sugar is ribose. In DNA (Deoxyribonucleic Acid), it is 2'-deoxyribose (lacking one oxygen atom at the 2' position).

A Nitrogenous Base: A flat, ring-like structure containing nitrogen. These are the "letters" of the genetic code.

A Phosphate Group: One or more phosphate groups attached to the 5' carbon of the sugar. This component provides the strong negative charge and the chemical energy required to link nucleotides together.

Visualizing the Structure: Imagine a nucleotide as a human body. The Base is the head (identity), the Sugar is the torso (the core structure), and the Phosphate is the arm extending out to hold hands with the next person in line.

2. The Nitrogenous Bases: Purines and Pyrimidines

The "identity" of a nucleotide is determined by its nitrogenous base. In classical biochemistry, we recognize five canonical bases, divided into two families based on their ring structure:

Purines (Double-Ring Structure):

Adenine (A): The metabolic powerhouse base.

Guanine (G): Crucial for G-protein signaling and structural stability.

Mnemonic: Pure As Gold (Purines = Adenine, Guanine).

Pyrimidines (Single-Ring Structure):

Cytosine (C): Found in both DNA and RNA.

Thymine (T): Found primarily in DNA.

Uracil (U): Found primarily in RNA (replaces Thymine).

Mnemonic: Cut The Py (Cytosine, Uracil, Thymine = Pyrimidines).

The "Expanded Alphabet" – A 2026 Perspective

As of 2026, we must acknowledge that the "four-letter" limit (A, T, C, G) is no longer absolute. Synthetic biology has successfully integrated Non-Canonical Nucleotides into living systems.

Hachimoji DNA: Scientists have engineered an eight-letter genetic system (adding bases Z, P, S, B). These synthetic nucleotides form stable hydrogen bonds and can be transcribed into RNA.

Why does this matter? It proves that the chemistry of life on Earth is not the only solution for information storage, opening doors for high-density DNA data storage and the search for extraterrestrial life with alternative biochemistries.

3. Functions of Nucleotides

While their role in DNA/RNA is famous, nucleotides are the "multitaskers" of the cell.

Genetic Information Storage: Polymerization of nucleotides creates the DNA double helix.

Chemical Energy Currency: Adenosine Triphosphate (ATP) is the universal energy coin. The breaking of its high-energy phosphoanhydride bonds powers muscle contraction, nerve impulses, and biosynthesis. GTP (Guanosine Triphosphate) powers protein synthesis.

Cellular Signaling: Cyclic AMP (cAMP) acts as a "second messenger." When a hormone (like adrenaline) hits a cell surface, it triggers a burst of cAMP inside, telling the cell to panic and mobilize energy.

Enzyme Cofactors: Many metabolic helpers (Coenzyme A, NAD+, FAD) contain nucleotide structures within them.

4. Nucleotide Synthesis: Making the Bricks

Cells have two strategies to acquire nucleotides:

De Novo Synthesis: "From scratch." The cell builds the ring structures atom-by-atom from simple amino acids (glutamine, glycine, aspartate) and CO2. This is metabolically expensive.

Salvage Pathways: "Recycling." The cell rescues free bases released during DNA/RNA degradation and reattaches them to a sugar-phosphate backbone.

Clinical Note: Defects in the salvage pathway lead to diseases like Lesch-Nyhan Syndrome, where uric acid accumulates, causing severe gout and neurological issues.

Part II: The Central Dogma – The Flow of Intelligence
Getty Images
1. The Classical Framework

Proposed by Francis Crick in 1958, the Central Dogma describes the directional flow of genetic information. In its simplest form, it is stated as:

DNA→RNA→Protein

This dogma dictates that:

DNA makes copies of itself (Replication).

DNA is read to make RNA (Transcription).

RNA is read to make Proteins (Translation).

However, in 2026, we view this not as a rigid rule, but as a "regulatory framework" with significant flexibility.
2. Replication: Preserving the Archive

Replication is the process where the entire genome is duplicated before cell division. It is semi-conservative, meaning each new DNA helix contains one old strand and one newly synthesized strand.

The Key Player: DNA Polymerase. This enzyme is the "typist." It reads the existing DNA strand and adds complementary nucleotides (A pairs with T, C pairs with G).

Fidelity: The error rate is incredibly low (1 in 10 billion bases) thanks to "proofreading" mechanisms.

3. Transcription: The Messenger

Transcription is the transcription of the "Master Blueprint" (DNA) into a portable "Working Copy" (mRNA).

The Process: RNA Polymerase unwinds a section of DNA and builds a single-stranded RNA molecule using Uracil (U) instead of Thymine (T).

The Promoter: This is the "Start Here" sign on the DNA that tells the enzyme where to begin.

2026 Insight: The Epitranscriptome (The "Fifth" Base)

Recent breakthroughs (2024-2026) have highlighted Epitranscriptomics. We used to think the mRNA was just a passive copy. We now know that after RNA is made, the cell chemically modifies it.

m6A Modification: The addition of a methyl group to Adenine in RNA affects how long the RNA lives and how efficiently it is translated.

Therapeutic Target: In 2026, drugs targeting METTL3 (the enzyme that adds these modifications) are in advanced clinical trials for treating leukemia and solid tumors. By blocking this modification, we can "starve" cancer cells of the proteins they need to grow.

4. Translation: The Factory Floor

Translation is the conversion of the nucleic acid language (nucleotides) into the protein language (amino acids).

The Machine: The Ribosome. This is a massive molecular factory made of rRNA and proteins.

The Key: tRNA (Transfer RNA). tRNAs are the "translators." One end holds a specific amino acid, and the other end has an "anticodon" that matches the code on the mRNA.

The Code: The genetic code is read in triplets called Codons.

AUG = Start (Methionine)

UAA, UAG, UGA = Stop.

5. Updates to the Dogma: Exceptions and Expansions

The "DNA → RNA → Protein" flow is not the only path. The 2026 syllabus emphasizes the "Reverse" flows:

Reverse Transcription (RNA → DNA):

Retroviruses (like HIV) use an enzyme called Reverse Transcriptase to turn their RNA genome back into DNA to hide in the host's genome.

Biotech Application: This mechanism is the basis for RT-PCR, the diagnostic gold standard (used in COVID-19 testing and modern viral load monitoring).

RNA Editing (RNA → Altered RNA):

Enzymes like ADAR can change an 'A' to an 'I' (Inosine) in the mRNA. This means the protein produced is different from what the DNA predicted. The cell effectively "edits the email" after it has been sent but before it is read.

Prions (Protein → Protein):

Prions are misfolded proteins that force other normal proteins to misfold. This represents a transfer of structural information from protein to protein without nucleic acids (e.g., Mad Cow Disease).

CRISPR and Prime Editing (RNA → DNA Modification):

Modern gene editing uses RNA guides to locate DNA sequences and modify them. In 2025/2026, Prime Editing allows us to "search and replace" DNA text with incredible precision, effectively rewriting the source code of the dogma.

Conclusion

The study of nucleotides and the Central Dogma is the study of biological continuity. From the simple purine and pyrimidine rings evolved a system of information storage so robust it has survived billions of years of evolution.

1. Introduction: The Molecular Choreography of Life

Welcome to the advanced module on nucleic acid chemistry. If you were studying this topic a decade ago, you might have viewed DNA as a static library of information and proteins as the mere workers that read it. Today, in 2026, we understand that this view is archaic. The reality of the cell is a chaotic, beautiful, and highly regulated dance where nucleic acids and proteins are rarely ever alone; they are locked in intimate, dynamic embraces called nucleoproteins.

This module will dissect the chemical anatomy of these complexes, stripping away the mystery to reveal the electrostatic engines that drive life. We will move beyond the simple "Watson-Crick" double helix to explore the wilder side of genetics—the knotty G-quadruplexes, the self-folding RNA origami that requires no protein scaffold, and the cutting-edge therapeutics that are currently redefining modern medicine. We are not just looking at molecules; we are looking at the machinery of existence.
2. Nucleoproteins: The Structural Gatekeepers

The Chemical Marriage of Opposites At its core, a nucleoprotein is a testament to the power of electrochemistry. It is a conjugated protein, a hybrid molecule consisting of a protein linked to a nucleic acid prosthetic group. But what glues them together? It is rarely a covalent bond. Instead, it is a salt-like attraction, a magnetic pull between opposites. The nucleic acid backbone is lined with phosphate groups (PO43−), rendering it profoundly negatively charged (polyanionic). To neutralize and package this charged cable, the cell employs proteins rich in basic amino acids—specifically Arginine and Lysine. These amino acids carry positive charges at physiological pH, allowing them to bind tightly to the phosphate backbone through electrostatic interactions and hydrogen bonding.

Significance: Why Package the Genome? Imagine trying to stuff a 2-meter-long thread into a thimble without it tangling. That is the challenge of the human nucleus. Nucleoproteins are the solution.

Histones (The Spools): The most famous example is the nucleosome. Here, DNA wraps 1.65 times around an octamer of histone proteins (H2A, H2B, H3, H4). This isn't just for storage; it's a control panel. By chemically modifying these histone tails (methylation, acetylation), the cell can "hide" genes from reading machinery or expose them.

Ribosomes (The Factories): The ribosome is perhaps the most complex ribonucleoprotein (RNP). It is a massive machine where ribosomal RNA (rRNA) acts as the catalyst—the ribozyme—while the proteins largely serve as structural scaffolding to keep the RNA stable.

Telomerase: This RNP protects the ends of our chromosomes, acting as a cellular clock.

2026 Perspective: The AI Revolution in Structural Biology We must acknowledge the massive leap occurring right now. Following the Nobel-winning work on AlphaFold (recognized in 2024), we can now predict the structure of these nucleoprotein complexes with near-atomic accuracy without needing decades of crystallography.

Current research in 2025-2026 has shifted from just "solving structures" to designing them. We are seeing the creation of "de novo" nucleoproteins—synthetic complexes designed by AI that can perform functions nature never intended, such as artificial viral capsids for drug delivery.

3. Deoxyribonucleic Acid (DNA): The Shapeshifting Archive

The Classical Structure (B-DNA) You know the classic staircase. Two antiparallel strands of polydeoxyribonucleotides twisted into a right-handed double helix. The chemical backbone is a repeating unit of deoxyribose sugar linked by 3′ −5′ phosphodiester bonds. Inside this hydrophilic protective cage lie the hydrophobic nitrogenous bases: Adenine (A), Guanine (G), Cytosine (C), and Thymine (T).

They pair with exquisite specificity: A with T (2 hydrogen bonds) and G with C (3 hydrogen bonds). This "base stacking" provides stability, creating a hydrophobic core that excludes water. This is the B-form DNA, the standard wet-lab structure. But if you dry it out, it crunches into the wider A-form. If you have a sequence rich in alternating GCGCGC, it can flip into a jagged, left-handed zig-zag called Z-DNA.

Beyond the Helix: The 2026 Frontier (G-Quadruplexes & i-Motifs) This is where standard textbooks fall short. In 2026, we know the genome is not just a smooth highway; it is full of speed bumps and knots that regulate traffic.

G-Quadruplexes (G4s): In guanine-rich regions (like telomeres and oncogene promoters), DNA can fold into a four-stranded knot. Four guanines arrange themselves in a square planar plate, stabilized by a central potassium ion (K+). These G4 structures act as "on/off" switches for cancer genes like c-Myc.

i-Motifs: On the complementary strand of a G4, cytosine-rich regions can form intercalated structures called i-motifs, which are pH-dependent.

Significance: Recent 2025 studies have shown that these structures are not accidents; they are recruited by the cell to control the speed of replication. Drugs that stabilize these "knots" are currently in Phase III clinical trials as novel chemotherapies, physically blocking cancer cells from accessing their own DNA.

4. Ribonucleic Acid (RNA): The Architect and The Tool

Chemical Distinctions RNA is often cast as DNA's unstable cousin, but chemically, it is the more versatile molecule.

The Sugar: It uses ribose, which has a hydroxyl group (-OH) at the 2' carbon. This extra oxygen makes RNA chemically more reactive and prone to hydrolysis (breaking down) in alkaline conditions. It is a feature, not a bug—RNA is meant to be transient.

The Base: Uracil (U) replaces Thymine. Uracil is energetically cheaper to produce for the cell.

The Shape: RNA is typically single-stranded, which allows it to fold back on itself like molecular origami, forming hairpins, loops, and pseudoknots.

The Functional Spectrum

mRNA (Messenger): The script carrier.

tRNA (Transfer): The physical adapter that translates genetic code into amino acids.

rRNA (Ribosomal): The catalytic heart of protein synthesis.

lncRNA (Long Non-Coding): Regulatory strands that don't make protein but can silence entire chromosomes (like the X-chromosome inactivation).

2026 Breakthrough: "Naked" RNA Architectures A pivotal discovery in mid-2025 by researchers at Stanford and SLAC upended the dogma that RNA needs proteins to form complex shapes. They discovered "protein-free" RNA complexes in bacteria—massive, symmetrical, multi-stranded RNA cages that assemble without any helper proteins. These "extravagant" shapes suggest that RNA is capable of far more structural independence than we realized. This has massive implications for synthetic biology: we are now trying to engineer RNA-only nanobots that can deliver drugs without triggering the immune system's anti-protein alarms.

Therapeutic Evolution: The Post-Vax Era By 2026, the mRNA technology popularized by COVID-19 vaccines has matured into circular RNA (circRNA) therapeutics. Unlike linear mRNA, which is chewed up by enzymes from the ends, circRNA is a continuous loop. It is infinitely more stable. We are seeing a surge in circRNA treatments for genetic diseases (like Huntington's) because a single dose can last for weeks rather than hours. Furthermore, RNA editing (using ADAR enzymes to fix mutations in the RNA without touching the DNA) is becoming a safer alternative to CRISPR, as it is reversible and carries no risk of permanent off-target genomic damage.

Conclusion: The Fluid Genome

To summarize this module, you must stop visualizing nucleic acids as static strings of letters. They are dynamic, breathing 3D entities. Whether it is the DNA double helix knotting itself into a G-quadruplex to stop a cancer cell, or a ring of circular RNA persisting in the cytoplasm to correct a genetic defect, these molecules are defined by their structure. Nucleoproteins are the mediators of this structure, the handlers that ensure the code is preserved, read, and regulated.

Your Takeaway Assignment: Consider the chemical difference between the 2' deoxyribose in DNA and the ribose in RNA. Why did nature choose the more stable (less reactive) sugar for the permanent storage (DNA) and the reactive sugar for the working copy (RNA)? The answer lies in the "OH" group—one oxygen atom that dictates the difference between a fleeting message and an eternal archive.

HEMOGLOBIN CHEMISTRY

Introduction: The Red River and the Chemical Factory

Welcome to this comprehensive exploration of one of the most elegant systems in the human body.

Think of this coursework as a story about logistics. We have a precious cargo (oxygen) that needs to be delivered to every cell. We have a vehicle (hemoglobin) designed perfectly for this task. We have a factory (the bone marrow) that builds the engine (heme) for that vehicle. And finally, we have a waste management and processing plant (the liver) that cleans up the mess when the vehicles break down.

In this deep dive, we will move through the molecular intricacies of hemoglobin, the volatile chemistry of making heme, and the diagnostic art of interpreting liver function. We will look at this through the lens of modern 2026 medical science, where genetic therapies and advanced diagnostics have reshaped how we view these classic biochemical pathways.

Part 1: Hemoglobin – The Molecular Lung

Hemoglobin (Hb) is not just a protein; it is a molecular machine. It moves, it breathes, and it changes shape in response to its environment. It is the primary vehicle for oxygen transport in the blood, found exclusively in red blood cells (erythrocytes).

1.1 Structure of Hemoglobin

To understand how hemoglobin works, we must look at its architecture. It is a globular protein with a quaternary structure, meaning it is built from multiple protein subunits sticking together.

The Globin Chains: Hemoglobin is a tetramer. This means it has four polypeptide chains. In a normal adult, the most common form (HbA) consists of two alpha (α) chains and two beta (β) chains. These chains are folded into tight helices, creating a protective pocket.

The Heme Group: Buried deep inside each of the four globin chains is a non-protein component called a "prosthetic group." This is Heme. Heme is a flat, ring-shaped molecule (a porphyrin ring). At the very center of this ring sits a single atom of Iron (Fe2+).

The Critical Connection: The iron atom is the star of the show. It is the magnet that holds the oxygen. Each iron atom can bind to one oxygen molecule (O2). Since there are four heme groups in one hemoglobin molecule, a single hemoglobin can carry four oxygen molecules.

1.2 Functional Dynamics: Allostery and Cooperativity

Hemoglobin is smarter than a simple storage box. It exhibits Cooperativity.

Imagine four people sitting in a car. If one door opens easily, it signals the other three doors to unlock. This is how hemoglobin binds oxygen.

When the first oxygen molecule binds to a heme group, it pulls the iron atom slightly.

This tug shifts the shape of the entire protein chain.

This shift forces the other three chains to open up, making it much easier for them to grab oxygen.

The T and R States:

T-State (Tense): This is the deoxygenated form. It is rigid and does not like oxygen. It releases oxygen to the tissues.

R-State (Relaxed): This is the oxygenated form. It is loose and loves oxygen. It grabs oxygen in the lungs.

The Oxygen Dissociation Curve: If you plot oxygen pressure against hemoglobin saturation, you get a Sigmoidal (S-shaped) curve, not a straight line. This S-shape proves that hemoglobin is greedy for oxygen in the lungs (where oxygen is high) and generous in the tissues (where oxygen is low).

Factors Affecting Function (The Bohr Effect): Hemoglobin knows where to drop off oxygen. It looks for metabolically active tissues (like exercising muscle). These tissues produce acid (H^+) and Carbon Dioxide (CO_2).

High CO_2 and Acid: Shift the curve to the right. Hemoglobin dumps oxygen.

2,3-BPG: This small molecule wedges into the hemoglobin and forces it to release oxygen. This is crucial for adapting to high altitudes.

1.3 Types of Hemoglobin

Not all hemoglobin is the same. Humans produce different models depending on their stage of development.

Hemoglobin A (HbA):

Structure: $\alpha_2\beta_2$

Status: The standard adult model. Makes up about 95-98% of hemoglobin in adults.

Hemoglobin A2 (HbA2):

Structure: α2δ2 (Alpha and Delta chains).

Status: A minor variant (2-3%). Elevated levels are a classic marker for Beta-Thalassemia trait.

Hemoglobin F (HbF - Fetal):

Structure: α2γ2 (Alpha and Gamma chains).

Status: The dominant form in the womb. HbF grabs oxygen much stronger than HbA. This allows the fetus to steal oxygen from the mother's blood across the placenta. It is usually replaced by HbA shortly after birth.

Hemoglobin S (Sickle Hemoglobin):

The Defect: A genetic mutation replaces Glutamic acid with Valine at position 6 of the beta chain.

The Result: When oxygen is low, HbS molecules stick together like long, rigid rods. This distorts the red blood cell into a "sickle" shape, causing blockages and pain.

Hemoglobin C (HbC):

The Defect: Glutamic acid is replaced by Lysine.

The Result: Causes mild anemia and crystals to form in the blood cells.

Part 2: Heme Synthesis & The Porphyrias

If hemoglobin is the car, Heme Synthesis is the manufacturing line for the engine. This process is chemically volatile. The intermediates (porphyrins) are highly reactive, particularly to light. If the assembly line breaks, toxic waste builds up.

2.1 The Heme Synthesis Pathway

This process happens in the Bone Marrow (85%) and the Liver. It is a relay race that jumps between the mitochondria and the cytosol of the cell.

The "Witch's Brew" Recipe:

The Start (Mitochondria): We start with two simple ingredients: Succinyl CoA (from the Krebs cycle) and Glycine (an amino acid). The enzyme ALA Synthase combines them to form ALA (Aminolevulinic Acid). This is the rate-limiting step—the traffic light that controls the speed of the whole pathway.

The Ring Building (Cytosol): ALA moves to the cytoplasm. Two ALA molecules are glued together to form a ring precursor called Porphobilinogen (PBG).

The Assembly: Four PBG molecules are linked to form a linear chain, which is then cyclized into a large ring structure (Uroporphyrinogen).

The Modification: Side chains are trimmed and modified (Coproporphyrinogen).

The Finish (Mitochondria): The molecule jumps back into the mitochondria. The final enzyme, Ferrochelatase, inserts the Iron (Fe^{2+}) atom into the center of the ring.

Protoporphyrin IX + $Fe^{2+} \rightarrow$ Heme

2.2 Disorders of Heme Synthesis: Porphyrias

Porphyrias are a group of rare genetic disorders. They occur when one of the specific enzymes in the heme assembly line is defective.

Think of an assembly line where the 4th worker goes on strike. The work from the first three workers piles up. In heme synthesis, this "pile up" consists of porphyrins. Porphyrins are purple pigments that react to UV light and damage tissues.

Classification of Porphyrias:

A. Acute Porphyrias (The Neuro-Visceral Attack) These affect the nervous system.

Acute Intermittent Porphyria (AIP):

Defect: PBG Deaminase enzyme.

Symptoms: Severe abdominal pain, hallucinations, paranoia, and racing heart rate. The urine may turn dark reddish-brown (like port wine) when left in the sunlight because the excess PBG oxidizes.

Historical Note: This is the disease famously theorized to have caused the "madness" of King George III.

B. Cutaneous Porphyrias (The Skin Attack) These affect the skin, making it blistering and fragile in sunlight.

Porphyria Cutanea Tarda (PCT):

Defect: Uroporphyrinogen decarboxylase.

Symptoms: Blistering on the back of hands, hyperpigmentation, and excessive hair growth (hypertrichosis) on the face.

Triggers: Alcohol, iron overload, and Hepatitis C often trigger this in genetically susceptible people.

The Vampire Connection: Some historians argue that severe cutaneous porphyria contributed to vampire folklore. Sufferers were pale (anemic), avoided sunlight (photosensitivity), had receding gums making teeth look like fangs, and may have had excess hair growth.

Part 3: Jaundice & Liver Function Tests (LFTs)

Eventually, red blood cells die. They live for about 120 days. When they shatter, the hemoglobin spills out. The body must recycle the iron and safely dispose of the heme ring. This disposal process is what gives us the yellow color of Jaundice.

3.1 The Lifecycle of Bilirubin

Breakdown: In the spleen, macrophages eat old red blood cells. They strip the iron from the heme (to reuse it). The remaining ring is opened up to become Biliverdin (green), which is then reduced to Bilirubin (yellow-orange).

Transport: This bilirubin is toxic and not water-soluble. It is called Unconjugated Bilirubin. It hitches a ride on Albumin (a protein taxi) to the liver.

Conjugation (The Liver's Job): The liver takes this toxic bilirubin and adds a sugar molecule (glucuronic acid) to it. This turns it into Conjugated Bilirubin. It is now water-soluble and safe.

Excretion: The liver pumps conjugated bilirubin into the bile, which goes to the intestine. Bacteria turn it into urobilinogen (which makes pee yellow) and stercobilin (which makes poop brown).

3.2 Classification of Jaundice

Jaundice is the yellowing of skin and eyes (sclera) due to high bilirubin. By 2026 standards, we classify this based on where the traffic jam occurs.

1. Pre-Hepatic Jaundice (The Overload)

Cause: The problem is before the liver. Usually, massive destruction of red blood cells (Hemolysis).

Mechanism: The liver is working fine, but it is overwhelmed by the sheer volume of bilirubin arriving from the spleen.

Lab Findings: High Unconjugated Bilirubin. Normal liver enzymes. Urine is normal color (unconjugated bilirubin can't get into urine).

2. Hepatic Jaundice (The Factory Failure)

Cause: The problem is inside the liver. Viral Hepatitis, Alcohol, or Cirrhosis.

Mechanism: The liver cells (hepatocytes) are sick. They cannot conjugate bilirubin efficiently, or they leak conjugated bilirubin back into the blood.

Lab Findings: Mixed High Unconjugated and Conjugated Bilirubin. High liver enzymes (ALT/AST). Dark urine.

3. Post-Hepatic Jaundice (The Blockage)

Cause: The problem is after the liver. Gallstones or a tumor blocking the bile duct.

Mechanism: The liver conjugates the bilirubin perfectly, but it can't flow into the gut. It backs up into the blood.

Lab Findings: Very High Conjugated Bilirubin. Pale, clay-colored stools (no pigment getting to gut). Dark, tea-colored urine (water-soluble bilirubin leaks into kidneys). Intense itching (pruritus) from bile salts depositing in skin.

3.3 Liver Function Tests (LFTs): The Panel

In clinical practice, we don't just look at one number. We look at the pattern of enzymes.

A. Markers of Hepatocellular Injury (Cell Death) These enzymes live inside liver cells. When cells die, they leak out.

ALT (Alanine Transaminase): Very specific to the liver. High levels mean liver inflammation.

AST (Aspartate Transaminase): Found in liver, heart, and muscle. Less specific.

The Ratio: In alcoholic liver disease, AST is often double the ALT (2:1 ratio). In viral hepatitis, ALT is usually higher than AST.

B. Markers of Cholestasis (Blockage) These enzymes live in the lining of the bile ducts.

ALP (Alkaline Phosphatase): rises when bile ducts are blocked or inflamed. (Also produced by growing bones).

GGT (Gamma-glutamyl Transferase): This is the tie-breaker. If ALP is high, we check GGT. If GGT is also high, the problem is definitely the liver/bile ducts, not the bone. GGT is also highly sensitive to alcohol use.

C. Markers of Synthetic Function (True Liver Function) The enzymes above only tell us about damage. These tests tell us if the liver is actually working.

Albumin: The liver makes this protein. Low albumin means chronic liver failure (the factory has been shut down for a long time).

Prothrombin Time (PT/INR): The liver makes clotting factors. If the PT is prolonged (blood takes too long to clot), it is an early warning of acute liver failure.

Conclusion: The Biochemical Symphony

As we conclude this coursework, notice how these systems are inextricably linked. Hemoglobin relies on Heme. Heme relies on a delicate synthesis pathway that, if broken, leads to Porphyria. When Hemoglobin finishes its job, it becomes the waste product that constitutes Jaundice. The Liver sits at the center of it all—synthesizing, detoxifying, and regulating.

In 2026, our understanding has moved beyond just identifying these pathways. We now use gene editing (like CRISPR-Cas9) to fix the errors in the globin genes for Sickle Cell patients. We use elastography to scan the liver's stiffness without using a needle. Yet, the fundamental biochemistry remains the same timeless logic of life.

Summary Table: Jaundice Differentiation

Type	Pathology	Dominant Bilirubin	Urine Color	Stool Color	Key Enzyme
Pre-Hepatic	Hemolysis (RBC Breakdown)	Unconjugated	Normal	Normal/Dark	Normal LFTs
Hepatic	Hepatitis/Cirrhosis	Mixed	Dark	Normal	High ALT/AST
Post-Hepatic	Bile Duct Obstruction	Conjugated	Dark (Tea)	Pale (Clay)	High ALP/GGT

Part 1: The Biochemistry of Hemolysis

Introduction to Red Cell Survival

To understand hemolytic anemia, we must first appreciate the Red Blood Cell (RBC). It is a marvel of biological engineering. Lacking a nucleus or mitochondria, it is essentially a flexible bag filled with hemoglobin, designed to squeeze through capillaries smaller than its own diameter.

Normally, an RBC lives for about 120 days. It works hard. It travels miles through the vasculature, subjected to high pressure and oxidative stress. Eventually, its metabolic machinery wears out. The membrane becomes rigid. The spleen, acting as the body's quality control filter, identifies these senescent (old) cells and removes them.

Hemolysis occurs when this process happens too fast. The bone marrow, which is the factory for blood cells, tries to compensate. It ramps up production (reticulocytosis). But if the destruction rate exceeds the production rate, the result is Hemolytic Anemia.

Classification of Hemolytic Disorders

We generally classify these disorders based on where the defect lies. Think of it this way: Is the problem with the car (the RBC itself) or the road (the environment)?

Intracorpuscular Defects (The Car is Broken): The problem is inside the red cell. These are usually hereditary.

- Defects in Hemoglobin (Sickle Cell, Thalassemia).
- Defects in Enzymes (G6PD Deficiency).
- Defects in the Membrane (Hereditary Spherocytosis).

Extracorpuscular Defects (The Road is Bad): The RBC is born healthy, but something outside kills it.

- Antibodies attacking the cell (Autoimmune).
- Physical trauma (Heart valves shearing the cells).
  - Infections (Malaria).

Part 2: Hemoglobinopathies – A Deep Dive

The most complex and chemically fascinating causes of hemolysis are the Hemoglobinopathies. These are genetic defects in the structure or synthesis of hemoglobin.

1. Sickle Cell Anemia (SCA)

This is the classic example of a "point mutation" causing systemic havoc.

The Biochemical Defect: In 2026, we understand this at the atomic level. Normal adult hemoglobin (HbA) is made of two alpha and two beta chains ($\alpha 2\beta 2$). In Sickle Cell disease, there is a single nucleotide substitution in the β-globin gene. An adenine is swapped for thymine (GAG→GTG).

Result: The amino acid Glutamic acid (hydrophilic/water-loving) is replaced by Valine (hydrophobic/water-hating) at position 6.

The Molecular Consequence (The "Sticky Patch"): This change seems minor, but it is catastrophic. When the RBC is oxygenated, everything is fine. But when the RBC releases oxygen (deoxygenated state), that hydrophobic Valine pops out. It acts like a sticky patch. It seeks shelter from the water in the cell and latches onto a hydrophobic pocket of a nearby hemoglobin molecule.

This causes the hemoglobin molecules to stack up like Lego blocks. They form long, rigid, rope-like fibers (polymers). These fibers distort the cell into the characteristic "sickle" or crescent shape.

Clinical Manifestation:

Vaso-occlusion: These stiff, sickled cells cannot bend to fit through tiny capillaries. They get stuck. This blocks blood flow, causing intense pain (pain crises) and tissue death (infarction).

Chronic Hemolysis: The cell membrane is damaged by the constant sickling and unsickling. The spleen destroys these cells rapidly.

2026 Perspective: While hydroxyurea has been the standard for decades, gene-editing therapies (like CRISPR-Cas9 based treatments approved in the early 2020s) are now becoming more accessible clinical realities. These therapies work by reactivating Fetal Hemoglobin (HbF), which does not sickle and interferes with the polymerization of HbS.

2. Thalassemia Syndromes

If Sickle Cell is a problem of quality (bad protein), Thalassemia is a problem of quantity (not enough protein).

The Biochemical Defect: Hemoglobin needs a perfect 1:1 ratio of alpha chains to beta chains. In Thalassemia, the synthesis of one of these chains is reduced or absent.

α-Thalassemia: Deletion of alpha-globin genes.

β-Thalassemia: Mutations in the beta-globin gene (promoter mutations, splicing errors).

The Mechanism of Damage (Imbalance): This is a key concept. The problem isn't just that there is less hemoglobin (which causes small, pale cells). The real killer is the unpaired chains.

In β-Thalassemia, there are no beta chains, so alpha chains accumulate.

These free alpha chains are insoluble. They precipitate inside the cell, forming toxic "inclusion bodies."

These inclusions damage the cell membrane from the inside out. They trigger "ineffective erythropoiesis," meaning the red cells die in the bone marrow before they are even released.

Clinical Manifestation:

Skeletal Deformities: Because the bone marrow is desperate to make more blood, it expands. This causes thinning of the bone cortex and deformities, typically in the skull (hair-on-end appearance on X-ray) and face (chipmunk facies).

Iron Overload: This is the secondary killer. Due to frequent transfusions and increased gut absorption, iron builds up in the heart and liver. Chelation therapy is mandatory.

Part 3: Enzymopathies & Membrane Defects
Glucose-6-Phosphate Dehydrogenase (G6PD) Deficiency

This is the most common enzyme defect in humans.

The Biochemical Role: RBCs rely on glycolysis for energy. A side-pathway, the Hexose Monophosphate Shunt, produces a molecule called NADPH.

NADPH is vital. It keeps Glutathione in a reduced state.

Reduced Glutathione is the cell's antioxidant bodyguard. It neutralizes hydrogen peroxide and free radicals.

The Defect: Without G6PD, the cell cannot make NADPH. The bodyguard (Glutathione) fails. When the patient is exposed to oxidative stress (certain drugs, infections, or Fava beans), hemoglobin gets oxidized. It turns into a precipitate called Heinz Bodies.

The Bite Cell: When these cells pass through the spleen, the splenic macrophages "bite" out the Heinz bodies, leaving a distinct "bite cell" shape.

Hereditary Spherocytosis

This is a structural engineering failure.

Defect: Mutations in proteins that tether the membrane to the internal skeleton (Spectrin, Ankyrin, Band 3).

Result: The membrane peels off in tiny vesicles. The cell loses surface area. It becomes a sphere (sphere = minimum surface area for a given volume).

Fate: Spheres are not flexible. They get trapped in the spleen and destroyed.

Part 4: Bilirubin – Synthesis, Types, and Fate

When these red cells are destroyed (hemolysis), they release hemoglobin. The body must clean up this mess. The result of this cleanup is Bilirubin.

1. Synthesis of Bilirubin

This is a catabolic (breakdown) pathway. It happens primarily in the macrophages of the Reticuloendothelial System (RES), mostly in the spleen.

Step A: Heme Ring Opening The hemoglobin is split into Heme and Globin. The Globin is recycled into amino acids. The Heme (the iron-containing ring) is the problem.

Enzyme: Heme Oxygenase.

Reaction: It cuts the heme ring open. This releases the iron (recycled) and Carbon Monoxide (CO). The remaining linear molecule is green. It is called Biliverdin.

Step B: Reduction

Enzyme: Biliverdin Reductase.

Reaction: The green Biliverdin is reduced to an orange-yellow pigment. This is Bilirubin.

2. Transport (The Taxi Ride)

The bilirubin formed in the spleen is Unconjugated Bilirubin (UCB).

Characteristics: It is hydrophobic (lipid-soluble). It cannot dissolve in blood. It is toxic to the brain.

The Solution: It binds tightly to Albumin, the main transport protein in the blood. Albumin carries it to the liver.

3. Hepatic Uptake and Conjugation

The liver is the processing plant.

Uptake: The hepatocyte (liver cell) takes the bilirubin from albumin.

Conjugation: To excrete bilirubin, the liver must make it water-soluble. It does this by gluing sugar molecules to it.

Enzyme: UDP-Glucuronosyltransferase (UGT1A1).

Reaction: Bilirubin + Glucuronic Acid → Conjugated Bilirubin (Bilirubin Diglucuronide).

Result: This "Direct" bilirubin is now water-soluble and non-toxic.

4. Excretion and Fate

The conjugated bilirubin is pumped into the bile ducts, stored in the gallbladder, and eventually released into the small intestine.

In the Intestine: Bacteria take over. Bacterial enzymes remove the glucuronic acid and reduce the bilirubin into colorless compounds called Urobilinogens.

Three Fates of Urobilinogen:

Excretion in Stool (Major Pathway): Most is oxidized to Stercobilin. This gives feces its characteristic brown color.

Enterohepatic Circulation: Some is reabsorbed into the blood and returned to the liver to be re-excreted.

Renal Excretion: A tiny fraction bypasses the liver, goes to the kidneys, and is excreted as Urobilin. This gives urine its yellow color.

Part 5: Clinical Correlation - Jaundice

Understanding the biochemistry allows us to diagnose the type of Jaundice (yellowing of skin/eyes) based on which type of bilirubin is elevated.

Pre-Hepatic Jaundice (Hemolytic):

Cause: Massive hemolysis (e.g., Sickle Cell crisis). The liver is working fine, but it is overwhelmed by the amount of heme arriving.

Lab Findings: High Unconjugated Bilirubin. Urine is normal color (because UCB cannot pass into urine), but stool is dark brown (excess Stercobilin).

Hepatic Jaundice:

Cause: Liver damage (Hepatitis, Cirrhosis). The factory is broken. It cannot conjugate or excrete effectively.

Lab Findings: Mixed High Unconjugated and Conjugated Bilirubin.

Post-Hepatic Jaundice (Obstructive):

Cause: A gallstone or tumor blocks the bile duct.

Lab Findings: High Conjugated Bilirubin. It backs up into the blood.

Signs: Dark urine (Conjugated bilirubin is water-soluble and enters urine). Pale/Clay-colored stools (No bilirubin gets to the gut to make Stercobilin).

Conclusion

The study of hemolytic anemia and bilirubin is a study of balance. It highlights the biochemical elegance of the human body. We see how a single amino acid change in Sickle Cell Anemia can alter the physical properties of blood. We see how the body possesses complex recycling systems to handle the toxic byproducts of heme degradation.

From the molecular precision of the G6PD enzyme to the macroscopic filtering of the spleen, these pathways represent a critical intersection of genetics, biochemistry, and physiology. As we move through 2026, our ability to manipulate these pathways through gene therapy and precision medicine continues to evolve, turning fatal genetic defects into manageable, or even curable, conditions.

This biochemical narrative confirms that structure determines function. When structure fails, pathology begins.

VITAMINS

1. Introduction: The Spark Plugs of Life

In the vast, interconnected machinery of the human body, macronutrients—carbohydrates, lipids, and proteins—are the fuel and the chassis. They provide the bulk energy and the structural framework. However, without vitamins, this machine would simply sit idle. Vitamins are the "spark plugs" of biochemistry; they are the organic compounds required in minute quantities to catalyze the metabolic reactions that sustain life.

As we stand here in 2026, our understanding of vitamins has evolved from viewing them merely as safeguards against deficiency diseases (like scurvy or rickets) to recognizing them as potent genomic regulators and immune modulators. We now understand that vitamins do not just prevent illness; they optimize genetic expression.

This coursework explores the biochemical architecture of vitamins, distinguishing their classes, and providing a deep-dive analysis into four critical players: Vitamin B12, Folic Acid, Vitamin C, and Vitamin D.

2. General Overview: The Biochemical Classification

Vitamins are distinct from other nutrients because they are not catabolized for energy (calories) but rather function primarily as co-enzymes or hormones.

2.1 The Solubility Divide

The solubility of a vitamin determines its absorption, transport, storage, and excretion. This is the fundamental divide in vitamin biochemistry.

Fat-Soluble Vitamins (A, D, E, K):

Absorption: Requires dietary fat and bile salts (micelle formation).

Storage: Stored in the liver and adipose tissue. This storage capacity means daily intake is less critical, but toxicity (hypervitaminosis) is a real risk.

Excretion: Fecal (via bile).

Water-Soluble Vitamins (B-Complex, C):

Absorption: Simple diffusion or carrier-mediated transport.

Storage: Minimal storage (except for B12). The body flushes excess through the kidneys.

Excretion: Urine. Toxicity is rare, but deficiency can occur rapidly (within weeks).

3. Deep Dive Analysis: Selected Vitamins

We will now transition to a rigorous examination of the specific vitamins requested.
3.1 Vitamin B12 (Cobalamin): The Cobalt Key

Vitamin B12 is arguably the most chemically complex of all vitamins. In 2026, we view B12 not just as an anemia preventer, but as a critical protector of the neural architecture.

Structure: B12 is a corrinoid. Its core structure resembles the heme found in hemoglobin, but with two crucial differences:

The central metal ion is Cobalt (Co), not iron.

The nitrogen-containing rings are linked directly, without a bridging carbon (corrin ring vs. porphyrin ring).

Forms: Cyanocobalamin (supplement), Methylcobalamin (active cytosolic form), and Adenosylcobalamin (active mitochondrial form).

Sources: B12 is synthesized exclusively by microorganisms. Humans obtain it solely from animal products: liver, clams, red meat, eggs, and dairy. Vegans are at 100% risk of deficiency without supplementation.

Functions: B12 acts as a cofactor for only two enzymes in the human body, yet these two govern life and death:

Methionine Synthase: Converts Homocysteine → Methionine. This reaction is vital for DNA methylation (epigenetics).

Methylmalonyl-CoA Mutase: Converts Methylmalonyl-CoA → Succinyl-CoA. This allows odd-chain fatty acids to enter the Krebs cycle. Without this, abnormal fatty acids accumulate in neuronal membranes (demyelination).

The "Methyl Trap" (2026 Biochemical Insight): You cannot discuss B12 without Folic Acid. If B12 is missing, the body's folate gets trapped in an unusable form (N5-methyl-THF). biochemical starvation ensues. This is the "Methyl Trap Hypothesis"—deficiency in B12 causes a functional deficiency in Folate.

Clinical Abnormalities:

Pernicious Anemia: An autoimmune destruction of Parietal Cells (which make Intrinsic Factor). Without Intrinsic Factor, B12 cannot be absorbed in the ileum.

Subacute Combined Degeneration: The hallmark B12 neuropathy. Demyelination of the dorsal columns of the spinal cord leads to loss of vibration sense, ataxia, and eventual paralysis.

Megaloblastic Anemia: Giant, immature red blood cells (MCV > 100 fL).

RDA (2026 Standard):

Adults: 2.4 mcg/day (Note: Needs increase significantly in pregnancy and for the elderly due to reduced gastric acid).

3.2 Folic Acid (Vitamin B9): The Architect of DNA

Structure: Folic acid is composed of three moieties:

A Pteridine ring.

Para-aminobenzoic acid (PABA).

Glutamic acid (polyglutamate tails trap it inside cells).

Functions (One-Carbon Metabolism): Think of Folate as a carrier of "carbon units." It grabs a single carbon atom (a methyl group, a formyl group) and pastes it onto other molecules. This is essential for:

DNA Synthesis: Making purines (Adenine, Guanine) and Thymidine. Rapidly dividing cells (bone marrow, fetus) crave folate.

Amino Acid Conversion: Serine to Glycine; Homocysteine to Methionine.

Sources: Derived from the Latin word folium (leaf). Rich sources include dark green leafy vegetables (spinach, kale), legumes, and fortified grains.

Clinical Abnormalities:

Neural Tube Defects (NTDs): If a mother is deficient in the first 28 days of pregnancy, the fetal spinal cord may not close (Spina Bifida, Anencephaly). This is why fortification is a public health mandate.

Megaloblastic Anemia: Identical to B12 deficiency anemia (large, fragile cells).

Glossitis: Inflammation of the tongue (smooth, red, "beefy" tongue).

RDA:

Adults: 400 mcg DFE (Dietary Folate Equivalents)/day.

Pregnancy: 600 mcg DFE/day.

3.3 Vitamin C (Ascorbic Acid): The Shield

Structure: A six-carbon lactone ring (γ-lactone). Structurally, it looks remarkably like glucose. Humans, guinea pigs, and fruit bats are among the few species that cannot synthesize it because we lack the enzyme L-gulonolactone oxidase.

Functions:

Collagen Synthesis: This is the most famous role. Vitamin C is a cofactor for the enzymes Prolyl Hydroxylase and Lysyl Hydroxylase. These enzymes add -OH groups to collagen strands, acting like "glue" that allows the strands to twist into a strong triple helix. Without C, collagen is unstable and falls apart.

Antioxidant: It scavenges free radicals in the aqueous (water) phase of cells, protecting DNA.

Iron Absorption: It reduces Ferric iron (Fe^{3+}) to Ferrous iron (Fe^{2+}), which is better absorbed by the gut.

Sources: Citrus fruits, kiwi, strawberries, bell peppers, and broccoli. Note: Vitamin C is heat-sensitive; cooking destroys it.

Clinical Abnormalities:

Scurvy: The breakdown of collagen.

Symptoms: Swollen/bleeding gums, petechiae (pinpoint hemorrhages under skin), poor wound healing, "corkscrew" hairs, and loose teeth.

Barlow's Disease: Infantile scurvy involving bone malformations.

RDA:

Men: 90 mg/day.

Women: 75 mg/day.

Smokers: Add 35 mg/day (due to increased oxidative stress).

3.4 Vitamin D (Calciferol): The Secosteroid Hormone

In 2026, we often argue that Vitamin D is not a vitamin at all—it is a pro-hormone.

Structure: It is a Secosteroid. This means it has the four-ring structure of a steroid (like cholesterol or testosterone), but one of the rings (Ring B) is broken open.

D2 (Ergocalciferol): From plants/fungi.

D3 (Cholecalciferol): From animal sources and sunlight (synthesized in skin from 7-dehydrocholesterol).

Metabolism (The Activation Pathway):

Skin: UV light converts cholesterol → Vitamin D3.

Liver: Hydroxylates it to 25(OH)D (Calcidiol - the storage form measured in blood tests).

Kidney: Hydroxylates it to 1,25(OH)2D (Calcitriol - the active hormone).

Functions:

Calcium Homeostasis: It acts on the intestines to increase Calcium absorption (via Calbindin protein) and on bones to mobilize calcium if blood levels drop.

Immune Modulation (2026 Insight): Vitamin D receptors (VDR) are found on macrophages and T-cells. Adequate D levels are now linked to reduced risk of autoimmune diseases (MS, Type 1 Diabetes) and better outcomes in viral respiratory infections.

Sources: Sunlight (UVB), fatty fish (salmon, mackerel), egg yolks, and fortified milk.

Clinical Abnormalities:

Rickets (Children): Soft, pliable bones leading to bow-legs and pigeon chest (rosary beads of ribs).
Osteomalacia (Adults): "Soft bones," bone pain, and muscle weakness.
Osteoporosis: Loss of bone mineral density in the elderly.

RDA:

Adults (19-70): 600 IU (15 mcg)/day.
Adults (>70): 800 IU (20 mcg)/day.
Note: Many biochemical experts in 2026 advocate for higher intakes (1000-2000 IU) to maximize non-skeletal (immune) benefits.

4. Summary Table: Clinical Abnormalities & RDA (2026 Verified)

Vitamin	Chemical Name	Key RDA (Adult)	Deficiency Disease	Key Clinical Signs
B12	Cobalamin	2.4 mcg	Pernicious Anemia	Neuropathy, Glossitis, Megaloblastic Anemia
B9	Folic Acid	400 mcg DFE	Neural Tube Defects	Megaloblastic Anemia, Spina Bifida (fetus)
C	Ascorbic Acid	75-90 mg	Scurvy	Bleeding gums, Corkscrew hair, Poor healing
D	Calciferol	600-800 IU	Rickets / Osteomalacia	Bone pain, Bow legs, Fracture risk

5. Conclusion: The Future of Micronutrients

As we conclude this biochemical analysis, it is evident that vitamins are the molecular custodians of our physiology. The "2026 Perspective" teaches us that RDAs are merely the baseline to prevent acute disease. The future of biochemistry lies in Nutrigenomics—understanding how genetic variations (like the MTHFR gene mutation in folate metabolism) dictate an individual's specific need for these vitamins.

MINERALS

Introduction: The Biochemical Currency of Life

Welcome to this deep dive into Mineral Metabolism. If we imagine proteins, fats, and carbohydrates as the "fuel" and "framework" of a building, minerals are the nuts, bolts, wiring, and spark plugs that make the house functional. They don't provide energy themselves (0 calories), yet without them, the energy machinery stops.

In this module, we are moving beyond simple memorization. We are looking at minerals as dynamic players in a high-stakes biochemical game. We will explore how the body aggressively guards its iron stores, how calcium decisions are made in milliseconds to keep your heart beating, and why a simple ion like fluoride changes the entire structural integrity of your teeth.

We will focus on the Macrominerals (required in large amounts) and the Trace Elements (vital micro-doses), incorporating the latest 2026 clinical standards and biochemical updates.

Part 1: The Heavyweights – Iron, Calcium, & Phosphorus

These three minerals are the foundation of physiological stability. Their regulation is so critical that the body has evolved complex hormonal feedback loops just to keep their blood levels within a razor-thin margin.

1. Iron (Fe): The Oxygen Logistics Manager

Iron is biologically expensive. Because it is so reactive (it rusts!), the body never lets it roam free. It is always chaperoned by proteins.

Functions

Oxygen Transport: About 65-70% of body iron is in hemoglobin, transporting oxygen from lungs to tissues. Another chunk is in myoglobin, holding oxygen in muscles for "fight or flight" bursts.

Electron Transfer: Iron is the "hot potato" handler in the Electron Transport Chain (cytochromes), shuttling electrons to generate ATP.

Enzymatic Reactions: It acts as a cofactor for enzymes involved in DNA synthesis and neurotransmitter production.

Sources & Bioavailability (2026 Context)

We distinguish between two types, a distinction that is crucial for modern plant-based diets:

Heme Iron (High Absorption): Found in animal flesh (meat, poultry, fish). The porphyrin ring protects it, allowing 15-35% absorption.

Non-Heme Iron (Low Absorption): Found in plants (spinach, lentils, fortified cereals). Only 2-20% is absorbed.

Bio-hack: Consuming Vitamin C (ascorbic acid) with plant sources reduces ferric iron (Fe^{3+}) to ferrous iron (Fe^{2+}), increasing absorption by 3-4x. Conversely, tannins (tea/coffee) and phytates (grains) block it.

RDA (Recommended Dietary Allowance)

Men & Post-menopausal Women: 8 mg/day.

Premenopausal Women: 18 mg/day (due to menstruation).

Pregnancy: 27 mg/day (a massive increase to support fetal blood volume).

Transport & Storage: The "Ferry and Vault" System

This is a sophisticated recycling system.

Absorption: Iron enters the enterocyte (gut cell) via the DMT1 transporter (only Fe^{2+} enters).

Export: It leaves the gut cell through a "doorway" protein called Ferroportin.

Transport: Once in the blood, it attaches to Transferrin. Think of Transferrin as a bus with two seats; it ferries iron safely to the bone marrow.

Storage: Excess iron is stored as Ferritin (a soluble, non-toxic cage) in the liver. If Ferritin overflows, iron clumps into Hemosiderin, which is insoluble and can damage tissues.

Clinical Importance

Iron Deficiency Anemia: The most common nutritional deficiency globally. Cells shrink (microcytic) and pale (hypochromic). Symptoms include fatigue, spoon-shaped nails (koilonychia), and pica (craving ice/dirt).

Hemochromatosis: A genetic disorder where the "brakes" on iron absorption fail. Iron overloads the liver and heart, leading to "bronze diabetes" (skin discoloration + pancreas damage).

2. Calcium (Ca^{2+}): The Signaling Architect

Calcium is unique because it serves two opposing roles: it is concrete (bones) and electricity (nerves).

Functions

Structural: 99% of calcium resides in bones and teeth as Hydroxyapatite crystals, providing rigidity.

Signaling: The remaining 1% in blood is strictly regulated. It controls muscle contraction (binding to troponin), nerve transmission, and blood clotting (Factor IV).

RDA (2026 Standards)

Adults (19-50): 1000 mg/day.

Women (50+) & Men (70+): 1200 mg/day (to combat bone density loss).

Teens: 1300 mg/day (peak bone mass building window).

Sources

Dairy: Milk, yogurt, cheese (high bioavailability).

Non-Dairy: Tofu (calcium-set), sardines (with bones), kale, and fortified plant milks. Note: Spinach has calcium, but it is bound by oxalates, making it unabsorbable.

Transport & Regulation

Calcium levels are controlled by a "thermostat" consisting of three hormones:

Parathyroid Hormone (PTH): If blood calcium drops, PTH signals bones to release calcium and kidneys to reabsorb it.

Vitamin D (Calcitriol): Increases calcium absorption in the gut. Without Vitamin D, you cannot absorb calcium, regardless of how much milk you drink.

Calcitonin: The antagonist. It tones down blood calcium by locking it into the bone (minor role in humans).

Clinical Importance

Hypocalcemia: Causes neuronal excitability. The classic sign is Tetany—involuntary muscle spasms. Doctors check for Chvostek's sign (tapping the cheek causes twitching) or Trousseau's sign (inflating a BP cuff causes hand spasms).

Osteoporosis: The "silent thief." Bone resorption exceeds formation, making bones porous and brittle.

3. Phosphorus (P): The Energy Backbone

Phosphorus is calcium's dance partner. They almost always move together or in opposition.
Functions

Energy Currency: It is the "P" in ATP (Adenosine Triphosphate). No phosphorus, no energy.

Genetic Structure: It forms the sugar-phosphate backbone of DNA and RNA.

Cell Membranes: Phospholipids make up the bilayer of every cell membrane.

Buffering: Phosphate buffers maintain blood pH balance.

RDA

Adults: 700 mg/day. (Deficiency is rare because it is abundant in most foods).

Sources

Found in protein-rich foods: meat, poultry, fish, eggs, nuts, and legumes. It is also heavily added to processed foods (sodas, additives), which has raised concerns in 2026 about kidney stress from too much phosphorus.

Clinical Importance: The Refeeding Syndrome

This is a critical concept for biochemistry students. If a patient is starving (anorexia or famine), their phosphate stores are depleted. If you feed them carbohydrates too quickly, insulin spikes. Insulin drives phosphate into the cells to make ATP for metabolism. This pulls the remaining phosphate out of the blood, causing severe Hypophosphatemia.

Result: Respiratory muscle failure (diaphragm weakness), cardiac arrhythmia, and death.

Lesson: "Start low and go slow" when feeding malnourished patients.

Part 2: The Protectors – Fluoride & Trace Minerals

While macrominerals build the house, trace minerals are the specialized workers maintaining the machinery. Even though we need them in microgram amounts, their absence is catastrophic.

1. Fluoride (F^-): The Enamel Shield

Fluoride is technically not "essential" for life (you won't die without it), but it is essential for dental health.
Biochemical Role

Tooth enamel is made of Hydroxyapatite ($Ca_{10}(PO_4)_6(OH)_2$).

The Swap: When fluoride is present, it replaces the Hydroxyl (OH^-) ion to form Fluorapatite ($Ca_{10}(PO_4)_6F_2$).

The Benefit: Fluorapatite is harder and much more resistant to acid attack (from bacteria) than the original enamel. It also actively remineralizes "soft spots" in teeth.

RDA (Adequate Intake)

Men: 4 mg/day.

Women: 3 mg/day.

Sources

Fluoridated water (public health standard).

Tea (tea leaves accumulate fluoride from soil).

Marine fish (with bones).

Clinical Importance

Dental Caries: Deficiency leads to weak enamel and cavities.

Fluorosis: Toxicity leads to chalky white patches or brown staining on teeth. It occurs if children swallow too much toothpaste while teeth are developing.

2. Other Essential Trace Minerals
A. Zinc (Zn): The Genetic Engineer

Function: Cofactor for over 300 enzymes. It stabilizes "Zinc Fingers"—protein structures that read DNA and regulate gene expression. It is vital for wound healing, sperm production, and taste perception.

RDA: 11 mg (Men), 8 mg (Women).

Sources: Oysters (highest source), beef, pumpkin seeds.

Clinical: Deficiency causes growth retardation in children, delayed wound healing, and hypogeusia (loss of taste).

B. Iodine (I): The Metabolic Thermostat

Function: Iodine has one job: it is incorporated into Thyroid Hormones (T3 and T4). These hormones set the Basal Metabolic Rate (BMR) for the entire body.

RDA: 150 mcg/day.

Sources: Iodized salt, seafood, seaweed (kelp).

Clinical:

Goiter: Without iodine, the thyroid gland enlarges, trying to trap more iodine.

Cretinism: Deficiency during pregnancy causes severe, irreversible mental disability in the infant.

C. Selenium (Se): The Antioxidant Bodyguard

Function: Component of Glutathione Peroxidase, an enzyme that neutralizes dangerous hydrogen peroxide in cells. It spares Vitamin E.

RDA: 55 mcg/day.

Sources: Brazil nuts (just 1-2 nuts provide the daily max), tuna, eggs.

Clinical: Deficiency is linked to Keshan disease (a cardiomyopathy found in soil-depleted areas).

D. Copper (Cu): The Cross-Linker

Function: Essential for iron absorption (ceruloplasmin) and for cross-linking collagen and elastin (via lysyl oxidase) to keep skin and blood vessels elastic.

RDA: 900 mcg/day.

Clinical: Menkes Disease (genetic copper deficiency) leads to "kinky hair" and neurodegeneration. Wilson's Disease (copper toxicity) leads to copper buildup in the liver and brain.

CARBOHYDRATE METABOLISM

Introduction: The Currency of Life

Welcome to the deep dive into Carbohydrate Metabolism. If the human body is a biological economy, carbohydrates are its cash flow, and metabolism is the banking system that manages it. We are not just talking about "burning sugar" here; we are discussing a sophisticated, tightly regulated network of chemical reactions that sustains consciousness, movement, and life itself.

As we stand here in 2026, our understanding of these pathways has moved beyond static textbook diagrams. We now see them as dynamic, personalized systems. For instance, recent data from Stanford Medicine suggests that "glucotypes" exist—meaning your metabolic reaction to a potato might be drastically different from your neighbor's, changing how we view the "universal" rules of digestion.

This coursework will guide you through the seven pillars of carbohydrate metabolism, from the moment a starch molecule touches your tongue to the complex dysregulation seen in diabetes.

1. Definitions: The Yin and Yang of Glucose

To understand metabolism, we must first define the two opposing forces that govern our energy states.

Glycolysis (The Breakdown) Glycolysis is the universal energy-harvesting pathway. Derived from the Greek glykys (sweet) and lysis (splitting), it is the sequence of ten enzyme-catalyzed reactions that converts glucose (a 6-

carbon molecule) into two molecules of pyruvate (a 3-carbon molecule).

The Vibe: It is an ancient pathway, occurring in the cytoplasm of nearly every living cell, from the bacteria in your gut to the neurons reading this sentence. It does not require oxygen, making it the primary energy source for anaerobic tissues like red blood cells and exercising muscle.

Gluconeogenesis (The Genesis) Gluconeogenesis is essentially the reverse—the synthesis of "new" glucose from non-carbohydrate precursors. When you sleep or fast, your supply of dietary glucose runs out. To keep your brain alive (which demands ~120g of glucose daily), your liver becomes a glucose factory.

The Precursors: It builds glucose from lactate (from exercising muscle), glycerol (from fat breakdown), and glucogenic amino acids (from protein).

The Location: It occurs primarily in the liver and, to a lesser extent, the kidney cortex. It is not just glycolysis run backward; it requires distinct enzymes to bypass the irreversible steps of glycolysis.

2. Digestion and Absorption: From Plate to Portal Vein

Imagine you have just eaten a complex meal—perhaps a bowl of rice (starch) and a sugary drink (sucrose). How does this fuel actually get into your engine?

Step 1: The Mouth (Salivary Phase) Digestion begins instantly. Salivary α -amylase acts as a molecular pair of scissors, randomly snipping the long α $(1 \rightarrow 4)$ glycosidic bonds of starch. However, this is brief. Once the food hits the acidic environment of the stomach, amylase is inactivated.

Step 2: The Small Intestine (The Real Work) The stomach is merely a holding tank. The real chemistry happens in the duodenum.

Pancreatic Amylase: The pancreas floods the intestine with a more potent amylase, breaking remaining starch down into maltose, maltotriose, and limit dextrins (branched chains).

Brush Border Enzymes: The final breakdown occurs right at the lining of the intestine (the brush border). Specific enzymes—maltase, sucrase, lactase, and isomaltase—act as the final checkpoint, converting these fragments into the "Big Three" monosaccharides: Glucose, Galactose, and Fructose.

Step 3: Absorption (The Gateway) Simple sugars cannot just float into the blood; they need VIP transport passes.

SGLT-1 (Sodium-Glucose Transporter 1): This is active transport. Glucose and galactose piggyback on sodium ions to enter the intestinal cell against their concentration gradient. It's like entering a crowded club by holding hands with a bouncer (sodium).

GLUT-5: Fructose takes a different door. It enters via facilitated diffusion using GLUT-5.

Step 4: Into the Portal Blood Once inside the intestinal cell, all three monosaccharides exit the back door via GLUT-2 and enter the hepatic portal vein. This is crucial: they don't go to the heart first; they go directly to the liver. The liver is the metabolic gatekeeper, deciding whether to store this energy or release it to the rest of the body.

3. Glycolysis: The Engine Room

Glycolysis is a ten-step drama played out in two acts: The Investment Phase (where we spend ATP) and the Payoff Phase (where we earn ATP).

Phase 1: Energy Investment (Priming the Pump)

Phosphorylation: Glucose is trapped inside the cell by adding a phosphate group.
Glucose+ATPHexokinaseGlucose-6-Phosphate+ADP

Note: In the liver, the enzyme is Glucokinase, which has a lower affinity, ensuring the liver only takes up glucose when blood sugar is high.

Isomerization: Glucose-6-P is rearranged into Fructose-6-P.

The Commitment Step: This is the most regulated step. Phosphofructokinase-1 (PFK-1) adds a second phosphate.
Fructose-6-P+ATPPFK-1Fructose-1,6-Bisphosphate

Regulation: High levels of ATP inhibit PFK-1 (signaling "we have enough energy"), while AMP activates it.

Phase 2: The Payoff (Harvesting) The 6-carbon molecule is split into two 3-carbon molecules (G3P and DHAP). From here, everything happens twice per glucose molecule.

Oxidation: G3P is oxidized, generating NADH (high-energy electron carrier).

ATP Generation: Two specific steps (catalyzed by Phosphoglycerate Kinase and Pyruvate Kinase) generate ATP directly. This is called "substrate-level phosphorylation."

The Fate of Pyruvate Pyruvate stands at a metabolic fork in the road. Its destiny depends on oxygen availability:

Aerobic (With Oxygen): Pyruvate enters the mitochondria, is converted to Acetyl-CoA by the Pyruvate Dehydrogenase Complex (PDH), and enters the Citric Acid Cycle. This yields massive energy (~30-32 ATP).

Anaerobic (No Oxygen): In sprinting muscles or red blood cells (which lack mitochondria), pyruvate is reduced to Lactate.

Pyruvate+NADHLactate DehydrogenaseLactate+NAD+

Why? This regenerates NAD+, allowing glycolysis to keep running even without oxygen.

4. The Citric Acid Cycle (TCA/Krebs Cycle)

If glycolysis is the engine, the TCA cycle is the turbocharger. It occurs in the mitochondrial matrix and is the "final common pathway" for the oxidation of carbs, fats, and proteins.

The Reactions (The Wheel turns)

Condensation: Acetyl-CoA (2 carbons) merges with Oxaloacetate (4 carbons) to form Citrate (6 carbons). Enzyme: Citrate Synthase.

Isomerization: Citrate is rearranged to Isocitrate.

First Decarboxylation: Isocitrate loses a carbon (CO2) and generates NADH. This forms a-Ketoglutarate.

Second Decarboxylation: a-Ketoglutarate loses another carbon (CO_2) and generates another NADH. We are now down to Succinyl-CoA (4 carbons).

Substrate Phosphorylation: The bond in Succinyl-CoA breaks, generating GTP (convertible to ATP).

Oxidation steps: Succinate is oxidized to Fumarate (producing $FADH_2$), then Malate, and finally back to Oxaloacetate (producing a final NADH).

Regulation: The Thermostat The cycle turns only when energy is low.

Citrate Synthase: Inhibited by ATP and Citrate (product inhibition).

Isocitrate Dehydrogenase: Activated by ADP (signaling low energy). Inhibited by ATP and NADH.

a-Ketoglutarate Dehydrogenase: Inhibited by Succinyl-CoA and NADH.

New Insight (2025): Recent research has highlighted how "oncometabolites" (mutated TCA intermediates like 2-hydroxyglutarate) can drive cancer progression, turning this life-giving cycle into a disease driver.
5. Glycogen Metabolism: The Storage Wars

Glucose is osmotically active—if you stored it as pure glucose, your cells would swell and burst. Instead, we polymerize it into Glycogen, a highly branched, safe storage form.

Glycogenesis (Making Glycogen) Occurs in the fed state (high insulin).

Glucose-6-P is converted to Glucose-1-P.

UDP-Glucose Pyrophosphorylase activates it to "UDP-Glucose" (high energy).

Glycogen Synthase adds the glucose to a growing chain (a-1,4 bonds).

Branching Enzyme creates branches (a-1,6 bonds) every 8-10 residues to increase solubility and speed of breakdown.

Glycogenolysis (Breaking it Down) Occurs in the fasting state (high glucagon/epinephrine).

Glycogen Phosphorylase nibbles the ends of the chains, releasing Glucose-1-P. Crucial Note: It uses phosphate, not water, to split the bond, saving energy.

Debranching Enzyme handles the branch points.

In the Liver: Glucose-6-Phosphatase removes the phosphate, releasing free glucose into the blood to feed the brain.

In Muscle: This enzyme is absent! Muscle glycogen is selfish—it can only be used by the muscle itself for energy.

Regulation: This is a masterpiece of phosphorylation cascades.

Insulin: Activates Protein Phosphatase-1, which dephosphorylates Glycogen Synthase (turning it ON) and Phosphorylase (turning it OFF). Result: Store fuel.

Glucagon/Epinephrine: Triggers cAMP, which activates kinases to phosphorylate both enzymes. Result: Synthase turns OFF, Phosphorylase turns ON. Result: Release fuel.

6. Hexose Monophosphate Shunt (HMP): The Side Hustle

While glycolysis produces energy (ATP), the HMP shunt (or Pentose Phosphate Pathway) produces currencies for construction and defense.

Purpose & Importance:

NADPH Production: This is distinct from NADH. NADPH is the "reducing power" used for:

Synthesizing fatty acids and steroids.

Antioxidant Defense: It recharges Glutathione, which neutralizes oxidative stress (Hydrogen Peroxide). Without NADPH, red blood cells die (hemolysis).

Ribose-5-Phosphate: The sugar backbone for DNA, RNA, and ATP synthesis.

The Reactions:

Oxidative Phase (Irreversible): Glucose-6-P is oxidized by Glucose-6-Phosphate Dehydrogenase (G6PD). This is the rate-limiting step and produces NADPH.

Non-Oxidative Phase (Reversible): Through a series of "carbon-swapping" reactions using enzymes like Transketolase and Transaldolase, the cell can convert ribose back into glycolytic intermediates (Fructose-6-P) if DNA synthesis isn't needed.

Clinical Context: G6PD Deficiency is the most common enzyme deficiency in the world. These individuals cannot produce enough NADPH. If they eat fava beans (which contain oxidizing agents) or take certain antimalarials, their red blood cells burst due to oxidative stress.

7. Blood Glucose & Diabetes Mellitus: When the System Fails

Normal Levels (Euglycemia):

Fasting: 70–99 mg/dL.

Post-prandial (after eating): <140 mg/dL. This tight range is maintained by the tug-of-war between Insulin (lowers sugar) and the Counter-regulatory hormones (Glucagon, Cortisol, Epinephrine, Growth Hormone).

Diabetes Mellitus (The Metabolic Derangement) Diabetes is not just "high sugar"; it is a state of "starvation in the midst of plenty."

Type 1 (Autoimmune): The immune system destroys pancreatic Beta-cells. Zero insulin.

Metabolic Chaos: Without insulin, cells cannot take up glucose. The body thinks it's starving. It breaks down fat (Lipolysis) and protein.

Diabetic Ketoacidosis (DKA): Massive fat breakdown floods the liver with Acetyl-CoA. Since the TCA cycle is stalled (due to low oxaloacetate), these Acetyl-CoA units form Ketone Bodies (Acetone, Acetoacetate, β-Hydroxybutyrate). The blood becomes acidic, leading to coma.

Type 2 (Insulin Resistance): Cells ignore the insulin signal.

Hyperglycemia: The liver keeps pumping out glucose (unsuppressed gluconeogenesis) while muscles refuse to take it up.

Dyslipidemia: The liver converts the excess sugar into VLDL (triglycerides), leading to fatty liver and atherosclerosis.

2026 Perspective: We are now moving toward "Precision Diabetology."

MASLD (formerly NAFLD): We now recognize that fatty liver is the hepatic manifestation of metabolic syndrome. It is a leading cause of liver failure.

Type 3 Diabetes: A growing body of 2024-2025 research links insulin resistance directly to Alzheimer's disease. The brain becomes "insulin resistant," leading to neurodegeneration.

Clinical Significance of Variations:

Hypoglycemia (<70 mg/dL): Dangerous because the brain relies almost exclusively on glucose. Symptoms: Tremors, confusion, coma.

Hyperglycemia (>180 mg/dL): Exceeds the kidney's threshold (Tm). Glucose spills into urine (Glycosuria), pulling water with it (Osmotic Diuresis).

Polyuria: Excessive urination.

Polydipsia: Excessive thirst (dehydration).

Polyphagia: Excessive hunger (cells are starving).

LIPID METABOLISM

Module Overview: The Energy Architecture of Lipids

Welcome to this advanced module on Lipid Metabolism. Today, we aren't just memorizing pathways; we are looking at the body's most sophisticated energy logistics system. Think of carbohydrates as the "cash in hand" for the body—easy to spend, quick to burn. Lipids, however, are the "gold bars" in the vault. They are dense, high-yield energy stores that require a specialized armored transport system to move around and a heavy-duty furnace to break down.

In this session, we will dissect the three critical pillars of this system:

The Logistics: How complex dietary fats are dismantled, shipped, and reassembled (Digestion & Absorption).

The Furnace: How we unlock the massive energy potential within fatty acids (Oxidation).

The Backup Generator: How the liver creates a "hybrid fuel" for the brain during starvation (Ketone Bodies).

Topic 1: Digestion and Absorption of Lipids

The Great Deconstruction and Reassembly

Dietary lipids are hydrophobic (water-fearing), yet they must navigate the aqueous environment of our digestive tract and blood. This presents a massive engineering challenge for the body. To solve it, we use a process I call "The Deconstruction-Reconstruction Protocol."

1. The Pre-Treatment (Mouth and Stomach)

Digestion begins the moment you chew. Lingual lipase (from glands behind the tongue) and gastric lipase (in the stomach) start the attack. They target short and medium-chain fatty acids (like those in milk), clipping them off the glycerol backbone.

Note: In adults, this contributes only about 10-20% of digestion, but in infants, this step is crucial for digesting breast milk.

2. The Main Event (Small Intestine)

When the acidic "chyme" (partially digested food) enters the duodenum, it triggers the release of two key agents:

Bile Salts: These are the "detergents" synthesized by the liver and stored in the gallbladder. They don't break chemical bonds; they break physics. They smash large fat globules into tiny microscopic droplets (emulsification). This increases the surface area for enzymes to work—like chopping a log into kindling so it burns faster.

Pancreatic Enzymes: The pancreas releases Pancreatic Lipase and Colipase. Lipase is the worker; Colipase is the anchor that holds Lipase onto the fat droplet so it doesn't slip off.

The Chemical Breakdown: Pancreatic lipase acts on Triacylglycerols (TAGs), snipping off the fatty acids at positions 1 and 3.
TriacylglycerolPancreatic Lipase2-Monoacylglycerol+2 Free Fatty Acids

3. The Smuggling Operation (Micelles)

The products (Free Fatty Acids, 2-Monoacylglycerol, Cholesterol) are still not water-soluble enough to swim to the gut wall. So, they form mixed micelles. Imagine these as tiny "ferry boats" made of bile salts with the fatty cargo hidden inside. They ferry the lipids through the "unstirred water layer" right up to the surface of the intestinal cells (enterocytes).

4. Intracellular Reconstruction (The Chylomicron)

Once inside the cell, the body does something counterintuitive. It rebuilds the fats it just broke down. The enterocyte re-esterifies the fatty acids back into Triacylglycerols. Why? Because you can't transport raw fatty acids in high concentrations without them being toxic.

These reformed fats are packaged into a massive lipoprotein particle called a Chylomicron.

The Cargo: TAGs (85%), Cholesterol esters.

The ID Tag: A specific protein called Apo B-48.

The Route: Chylomicrons are too big for blood capillaries. Instead, they enter the Lacteals (lymphatic vessels). They travel through the lymph and are dumped into the bloodstream near the heart (thoracic duct), bypassing the liver initially. This ensures muscle and adipose tissue get "first dibs" on the fuel.

Topic 2: Fatty Acid Oxidation

The Mitochondrial Power Plant

Once lipids are stored in adipose tissue, we need a way to retrieve them when energy is low (like during sleep or exercise). This is Beta-Oxidation (β-oxidation).

Step 1: Mobilization (The Wake-Up Call)

When blood sugar drops, hormones like Glucagon or Epinephrine hit the fat cells. This triggers Hormone Sensitive Lipase (HSL) to break down stored fat into Free Fatty Acids (FFA) and Glycerol. The Glycerol goes to the liver for gluconeogenesis; the FFAs hitch a ride on Albumin (the blood's taxi service) to reach tissues like muscle.

Step 2: Activation and Transport (The Security Check)

Fatty acids cannot just walk into the mitochondria where oxidation happens. They must be "tagged" and "escorted."

Activation: The fatty acid is attached to Coenzyme A by the enzyme Acyl-CoA Synthetase. This costs 2 ATP equivalents.

$$\text{Fatty Acid} + \text{ATP} + \text{CoA} \rightarrow \text{Acyl-CoA} + \text{AMP} + \text{PPi}$$

The Carnitine Shuttle: The inner mitochondrial membrane is impermeable to Acyl-CoA. The "Carnitine Shuttle" system swaps the CoA for Carnitine, moves it across, and swaps it back.

Rate Limiting Step: The enzyme CPT-1 (Carnitine Palmitoyltransferase I) controls this entry. It is inhibited by Malonyl-CoA (which is high when we are well-fed), preventing us from burning fat when we are actively building it.

Step 3: Beta-Oxidation (The Spiral Staircase)

Inside the mitochondrial matrix, the fatty acid undergoes a cyclic process. I call it a "spiral" because with every turn, the chain gets shorter by 2 carbons. Each cycle consists of four steps:

Oxidation (FAD linked): Creates a double bond. Yields 1.5 ATP.

Hydration: Adds water across the bond.

Oxidation (NAD+ linked): Converts hydroxyl to keto group. Yields 2.5 ATP.

Thiolysis: Cleaves off Acetyl-CoA.

The Yield: For a standard 16-carbon fatty acid (Palmitate):

We run the spiral 7 times.

We produce 8 Acetyl-CoA.

We produce 7 $FADH_2$ and 7 NADH.

The Acetyl-CoA then enters the Krebs Cycle for even more energy. The total net yield for one Palmitate is approximately 106 ATP (older texts say 129, but 106 is the modern P/O ratio adjusted value). Compare this to Glucose (30-32 ATP), and you see why fat is the gold standard for energy storage.

2026 Update: Metabolic Flexibility New research (published late 2025/early 2026) highlights that "Metabolic Flexibility"—the ability to switch cleanly between glucose oxidation (fed state) and fatty acid oxidation (fasted state)—is heavily regulated by circadian rhythms. A 2026 study in Cell Metabolism revealed that exposure to natural daylight during office hours significantly boosts this flexibility in Type 2 Diabetics, effectively "tuning" the mitochondria to switch to fat oxidation more efficiently during fasting windows.

Topic 3: Ketone Bodies (Synthesis & Utilization)

The Brain's Emergency Hybrid Fuel

The brain is a picky eater. It cannot use fatty acids because they are bound to albumin and cannot cross the Blood-Brain Barrier (BBB). During starvation or prolonged fasting, when glucose runs out, the body needs a workaround. Enter Ketone Bodies.

Synthesis (Ketogenesis)

This occurs exclusively in the Liver mitochondria. When fatty acid oxidation is running at high speed (e.g., starvation), the liver produces massive amounts of Acetyl-CoA. The Krebs cycle cannot handle this influx because its intermediates (like oxaloacetate) are being pulled away to make glucose. So, the excess Acetyl-CoA is diverted:

Condensation: 2 Acetyl-CoA form Acetoacetyl-CoA.

HMG-CoA Step: HMG-CoA Synthase creates HMG-CoA. (This is the rate-limiting step).

Cleavage: HMG-CoA Lyase breaks it into Acetoacetate (the first ketone body).

Conversion: Acetoacetate can be reduced to β-Hydroxybutyrate (BHB) or spontaneously decarboxylate to Acetone (which gives the "fruity breath" smell in ketoacidosis).

Utilization (Ketolysis)

The liver makes ketones but cannot use them (it lacks the enzyme Thiolase). Ketones are soluble in blood (no albumin needed). They travel to the brain, heart, and muscle.

BHB is converted back to Acetoacetate.

Acetoacetate is activated to Acetoacetyl-CoA by the enzyme Thiophorase (succinyl-CoA:3-ketoacid CoA transferase).

This is split into 2 Acetyl-CoA molecules, which enter the Krebs cycle to generate ATP.

Clinical & Modern Context (2026 Perspectives)

The BHB Shunt (New Discovery): We used to think BHB was just a fuel. However, research emerging in late 2024 and solidified in 2025 has identified the "BHB Shunt." An enzyme called CNDP2 can divert BHB to form BHB-amino acids (like BHB-Phenylalanine). These novel metabolites act as signaling molecules in the brain to suppress appetite. This explains why hunger often decreases during deep ketosis (fasting).

Ketoacidosis vs. Ketosis:

Nutritional Ketosis: Controlled, low levels (0.5 - 3 mM). Safe and adaptive.

Ketoacidosis (DKA): Uncontrolled, massive levels (>10-20 mM) seen in Type 1 Diabetes. The pH of the blood drops dangerously low because ketone bodies are acidic.

ELECTRON TRANSPORT CHAIN AND NEUROTRANSMITTERS

Part 1: The Electron Transport Chain (ETC) and ATP Synthesis

1.1 Introduction to Cellular Currency

Imagine standing inside a hydroelectric dam. You see massive turbines spinning, water rushing through gates, and electricity humming through wires. This is exactly what happens inside your cells, specifically within the mitochondria. But instead of water, we use electrons. Instead of concrete dams, we use biological membranes.

The Electron Transport Chain (ETC) is the culmination of cellular respiration. It is where the chemical energy stored in the food we eat—broken down through glycolysis and the Krebs cycle—is finally converted into ATP (Adenosine Triphosphate), the universal currency of biological energy.

Shutterstock
1.2 The Stage: Structure of the ETC

The ETC is located on the inner mitochondrial membrane. This membrane is folded into ridges called cristae to maximize surface area. It separates the mitochondrial matrix (the inside) from the intermembrane space (the outside). This separation is crucial. Without a sealed barrier, the battery cannot hold a charge.

The chain itself consists of four distinct protein complexes (labeled I through IV) embedded in the lipid bilayer, along with two mobile electron carriers: Ubiquinone (Coenzyme Q) and Cytochrome c.

Recent structural biology (as of 2026) emphasizes that these complexes are not just floating randomly. They often organize into "Supercomplexes" or Respirasomes. This clustering makes electron transfer more efficient, like organizing factory workers into a tight assembly line rather than having them shout across a large warehouse.

1.3 The Mechanism: Passing the Baton

The goal is simple: extract energy from electrons to pump protons (H+) out of the matrix. This creates a pressure gradient. Here is the step-by-step flow:

Complex I: NADH-CoQ Oxidoreductase

This is the entry point for electrons carried by NADH. Complex I is a massive "L-shaped" protein.

The Action: NADH donates two electrons to the complex. These electrons travel through a wire-like series of iron-sulfur clusters.

The Result: As the electrons move, they trigger a conformational change—a physical shape shift in the protein—that pumps 4 protons (H+) from the matrix into the intermembrane space.

The Handoff: The electrons are finally passed to Ubiquinone (Q), reducing it to Ubiquinol (QH2).

Complex II: Succinate-Q Reductase

This complex is unique because it is physically part of the Krebs Cycle. It takes electrons from FADH$_2$ (generated from succinate).

The Action: It passes electrons to Ubiquinone.

The Note: It does not pump protons. It just feeds electrons into the system. This explains why FADH$_2$ produces less ATP than NADH; it enters the chain "downstream" of the first pump.

Complex III: Q-Cytochrome c Oxidoreductase

Here, the reduced Ubiquinol (QH2) arrives carrying electrons.

The Q-Cycle: This is a sophisticated switching mechanism. Complex III takes electrons from QH2 and passes them to Cytochrome c.

The Result: During this transfer, 4 more protons are pumped into the intermembrane space.

The Carrier: Cytochrome c is a small, water-soluble protein that acts as a shuttle, ferrying electrons one by one to the final station.

Shutterstock

Complex IV: Cytochrome c Oxidase

This is the final destination.

The Action: Complex IV receives electrons from Cytochrome c. It holds onto them until it has enough to perform a critical reaction: reducing molecular Oxygen (O2).

The Chemistry:
$O2+4e-+4H+ \rightarrow 2H2O$

The Result: This is why we breathe. Oxygen is the "final electron acceptor." Without oxygen, the chain creates a

traffic jam, everything stops, and the cell suffocates.
Complex IV pumps 2 final protons across the membrane.

1.4 Synthesis of ATP: Chemiosmosis

By this point, we have built a massive reservoir of protons in the intermembrane space. This creates two forces:

Chemical Gradient: Difference in concentration (pH).

Electrical Gradient: Difference in charge (positive outside, negative inside).

Together, this is the Proton-Motive Force.
Complex V: ATP Synthase

This is arguably the most beautiful protein in nature. It is a rotary motor.

Structure: It has a rotor (F0) embedded in the membrane and a stator (F1) sticking into the matrix.

Function: Protons flow back into the matrix through the F0 subunit, driven by the gradient. This flow forces the central shaft of the protein to spin at incredible speeds (up to 9,000 RPM).

Synthesis: As the shaft rotates inside the F1 head, it physically crushes ADP and Phosphate (Pi) together to form ATP.

ADP+Pi+Energy (Proton flow)→ATP+H2O

This process is called Oxidative Phosphorylation. For every NADH, we generate roughly 2.5 ATP. For every FADH$_2$, we generate roughly 1.5 ATP.

Part 2: Neurotransmitters

2.1 Overview of Chemical Messaging

If the ETC is the power plant, neurotransmitters are the fiber-optic cables of the biological world. The nervous system runs on electricity (action potentials), but neurons don't usually touch each other. There is a gap called the synapse. To cross this gap, the electrical signal must be converted into a chemical signal. That chemical is a neurotransmitter.

2.2 Chemistry and Classification

Neurotransmitters are small molecules with diverse chemical roots. We categorize them based on their structure:

- Amino Acids: The workhorses of the brain.
  - Glutamate: The primary "go" signal (excitatory).
  - GABA (Gamma-aminobutyric acid): The primary "stop" signal (inhibitory).
  - Glycine: Inhibitory, mostly in the spinal cord.
- Monoamines (Biogenic Amines): The regulators of mood and attention.
- Catecholamines: Dopamine, Norepinephrine, Epinephrine (derived from tyrosine).

Indolamines: Serotonin (derived from tryptophan).

- Acetylcholine: The driver of muscle contraction and memory.

Neuropeptides: Larger molecules like endorphins and Substance P (pain signals).

2.3 Biosynthesis: The Assembly Line

Neurotransmitters are synthesized locally within the neuron. The synthesis pathways are tightly regulated enzymatic chains.

Example 1: The Dopamine Pathway

This is a classic example of "metabolic funneling."

Precursor: It starts with the amino acid Tyrosine (from diet).

Step 1: The enzyme Tyrosine Hydroxylase adds a hydroxyl group to form L-DOPA. This is the rate-limiting step—the bottleneck that controls how much dopamine is made.

Step 2: The enzyme DOPA Decarboxylase removes a carboxyl group (CO_2) to form Dopamine.

If the neuron needs Norepinephrine, it adds another step using Dopamine Beta-Hydroxylase. This illustrates the metabolic economy: the body modifies existing structures rather than building new ones from scratch.

Shutterstock

Example 2: Acetylcholine (ACh)

This synthesis is a marriage of sugar metabolism and fat metabolism.

Acetate: Derived from Acetyl-CoA (from the mitochondria/Krebs cycle).

Choline: Derived from lipids in the diet.

Enzyme: Choline Acetyltransferase fuses them together.

2.4 Mechanism of Action

How does the message get delivered?

Storage: Once made, neurotransmitters are packed into synaptic vesicles. They sit at the edge of the neuron terminal, waiting.

Release: When an electrical action potential hits the terminal, voltage-gated Calcium channels open. Calcium rushes in. This calcium triggers the vesicles to fuse with the membrane (exocytosis), spilling their contents into the synaptic gap.

Binding: The neurotransmitters swim across the gap and bind to receptors on the receiving cell.

The Two Types of Receptors

Ionotropic Receptors (Fast): These are direct gates. When the neurotransmitter binds, the channel pops open immediately. Ions rush in. This is fast, precise signaling (e.g., pulling your hand away from a hot stove).

Metabotropic Receptors (Slow/Modulatory): These are G-protein coupled receptors (GPCRs). When the neurotransmitter binds, it triggers a cascade of internal cellular messengers. This changes the "mood" of the cell, making it more or less sensitive to future signals. This is how memories and emotional states persist.

2.5 Termination: Cleaning the Slate

The signal must stop eventually, or the neuron would be permanently stuck "on."

Reuptake: Transporter pumps vacuum the neurotransmitter back into the sending neuron to be recycled (e.g., SSRI antidepressants work by blocking the serotonin vacuum).

Enzymatic Degradation: Enzymes chew up the neurotransmitter in the gap. For example, Acetylcholinesterase breaks down Acetylcholine so quickly that muscles can relax milliseconds after contracting.

2.6 Metabolic Role & Integration

Neurotransmitters are not just signals; they are deeply integrated into the body's general metabolism.

The Glutamate-Gamine Cycle: In the brain, glial cells (support cells) mop up excess Glutamate to prevent toxicity. They convert it to Glutamine (which is safe) and send it back to the neuron. This cycle consumes a significant portion of the brain's ATP.

Glycolysis Link: The synthesis of Glutamate and GABA is directly linked to the Krebs Cycle intermediates (a-ketoglutarate). This means if your brain runs out of glucose (energy), it might start cannibalizing its own neurotransmitter precursors, leading to confusion or coma.

Part 3: Conclusion and Future Perspectives (2026 Analysis)

3.1 The Convergence of Bioenergetics and Signaling

We often study the ETC and Neurotransmitters as separate chapters, but in 2026, we understand they are inextricably linked.

The production of ATP in the mitochondria is required to package neurotransmitters into vesicles and to run the pumps that clear them from the synapse. Conversely, neurotransmitters like Glutamate can stimulate mitochondria to speed up respiration.

3.2 New Frontiers

Current research is revealing that mitochondrial defects are often the root cause of "neurochemical" diseases. For instance, in Parkinson's disease, we now know that Complex I of the ETC often malfunctions specifically in dopamine neurons. This leads to an energy crisis that kills the cell.

Furthermore, we are seeing the rise of "Mitoneurotherapeutics"—drugs designed not just to target receptors on the surface of neurons, but to penetrate the mitochondria and stabilize the Electron Transport Chain directly.

Summary

From the sub-atomic flow of electrons down a protein wire to the complex burst of chemicals that allows you to read this sentence, life is a delicate balance of energy and information. The Electron Transport Chain provides the fuel; Neurotransmitters provide the code. Together, they form the biochemical basis of consciousness and animation.

PROTEIN METABOLISM

Module Introduction: The Body's Grand Recycling Plant

Welcome to this deep dive into Protein Metabolism. If carbohydrates are the fuel of the human body, proteins are the machinery, the scaffolding, and the communication network. But unlike a static building, this machinery is constantly being torn down and rebuilt. As of early 2026, our understanding of this process has shifted from viewing it as a simple "intake and output" system to recognizing it as a complex interplay between host enzymes, genetic programming, and—crucially—our gut microbiome.

In this module, we will explore the journey of a dietary protein from the moment it enters your system to its ultimate fate, whether that be building new muscle, becoming a neurotransmitter, or being detoxified and excreted. We will also examine what happens when this delicate machinery fails, looking at the very latest therapeutic breakthroughs for metabolic disorders as of late 2025 and early 2026.

1. Digestion and Absorption: Breaking Down the Complex

Dietary proteins are large, chemically complex polymers of amino acids linked by peptide bonds. For the body to utilize them, they must be dismantled into their individual components. Imagine trying to transport a Lego castle through a small doorway; you have to break it down into individual bricks first.

A. The Gastric Phase: The Acid Bath

The process begins in the stomach, which acts as a chemical mixing tank.

Hydrochloric Acid (HCl): Secreted by parietal cells, HCl does not break the peptide bonds directly but denatures the protein. It uncoils the complex 3D structures, making the peptide bonds accessible.

Pepsin: This is the primary proteolytic enzyme of the stomach. It is secreted as an inactive precursor called pepsinogen (a zymogen) to prevent it from digesting the stomach lining itself. Upon contact with HCl, it auto-catalyzes into active pepsin. Pepsin cleaves proteins into smaller polypeptides and oligopeptides, favoring bonds involving aromatic amino acids like phenylalanine and tyrosine.

B. The Pancreatic Phase: Precision Cutting

As the acidic chyme enters the small intestine (duodenum), it triggers the release of secretin and cholecystokinin (CCK). These hormones signal the pancreas to release a cocktail of powerful enzymes:

Trypsinogen & Chymotrypsinogen: Activated by enteropeptidase in the intestine to form Trypsin and Chymotrypsin. These continue chopping the polypeptides into smaller fragments.

Carboxypeptidases (A and B): These are exopeptidases, meaning they nibble amino acids off the "C-terminal" end of the chain one by one.

Elastase: Breaks down elastin and other structural proteins.

C. Intestinal Absorption: The Final Gatekeepers

By the time the mixture reaches the jejunum and ileum, we are left with free amino acids, dipeptides, and tripeptides.

Brush Border Enzymes: Enzymes like aminopeptidase sitting on the surface of intestinal cells finish the job.

Transport Mechanisms (2026 Update): Absorption is not passive; it requires energy. Sodium-dependent transporters (like the SLC7 family) drag amino acids into the cell against their concentration gradient.

Recent Insight: Research published in mid-2025 has highlighted the critical role of the LAT1 (SLC7A5) transporter not just in absorption, but as a regulator of insulin signaling. Dysregulation here is now being linked to the pathophysiology of diabetes, changing how we view "simple" absorption.

2026 Microbiome Breakthrough: Historically, we believed protein digestion was almost entirely a host process. However, a landmark study from NC State University (August 2025) has rewritten this chapter. We now know that the gut microbiome plays a massive role in digesting proteins that escape the small intestine. Specifically, the microbiome modifies glycans (sugar chains) attached to proteins, and the source of the protein (animal vs. plant) dictates which bacterial species thrive. This "second digestion" in the colon produces metabolites that can either boost immunity or release toxins, depending on your diet.

2. Amino Acid Reactions & Ammonia Metabolism

Once absorbed, amino acids enter the "Amino Acid Pool"—a circulating reserve available for protein synthesis, energy production, or conversion into specialized molecules.

A. General Reactions: The "Swap and Drop"

Most amino acids undergo two key reactions to be utilized for energy:

Transamination (The Swap):

The alpha-amino group is transferred to a keto acid (usually alpha-ketoglutarate).

Enzymes: Transaminases (or Aminotransferases) like ALT (Alanine Transaminase) and AST (Aspartate Transaminase).

Result: The amino acid becomes a keto acid (which can enter the Krebs cycle for energy), and the alpha-ketoglutarate becomes Glutamate. This funnels the nitrogen into one molecule (Glutamate), simplifying disposal.

Deamination (The Drop):

Now, that Glutamate must shed its nitrogen. This occurs via Oxidative Deamination, primarily in the liver.

Enzyme: Glutamate Dehydrogenase.

Result: Glutamate releases the amino group as free Ammonia (NH_3) and reverts to alpha-ketoglutarate.

B. Ammonia Metabolism: The Urea Cycle

Ammonia is highly toxic, especially to the brain. The body must convert it into Urea, a water-soluble and non-toxic compound, for excretion by the kidneys. This process, known as the Urea Cycle, occurs exclusively in the liver.

The 5 Steps of the Urea Cycle:

Formation of Carbamoyl Phosphate: Ammonia + CO2 + 2 ATP → Carbamoyl Phosphate. (Enzyme: CPS-1). This is the rate-limiting step.

Synthesis of Citrulline: Carbamoyl Phosphate + Ornithine → Citrulline.

Synthesis of Argininosuccinate: Citrulline + Aspartate → Argininosuccinate.

Cleavage: Argininosuccinate is split into Arginine and Fumarate. (Fumarate can enter the TCA cycle, linking protein and carb metabolism).

Formation of Urea: Arginine is hydrolyzed by Arginase to produce Urea and regenerate Ornithine.

2025-2026 Research Update - "The Pyrimidine Connection": New research from the Ben-Sahra Lab (published late 2024/2025) has uncovered a previously unknown link. They found that pyrimidine nucleotides (building blocks of DNA) act as phosphate donors to activate Vitamin B1, which in turn fuels the enzyme Pyruvate Dehydrogenase. This proves that protein/nucleotide metabolism is intimately tied to the TCA cycle's ability to burn carbs and fats. It's a major shift in biochemistry textbooks: protein metabolism isn't an island; it drives the central energy machinery.

3. Metabolism of Specific Amino Acids & Inborn Errors

When the genetic code for enzymes in these pathways contains errors, we get "Inborn Errors of Metabolism." These are often rare but devastating. However, 2026 is a year of hope, with new therapies moving from the lab to the clinic.

A. Phenylalanine & Tyrosine (The Aromatic Pathway)

Normal Pathway: Phenylalanine is converted to Tyrosine by the enzyme Phenylalanine Hydroxylase (PAH). Tyrosine is then used to make dopamine, melanin, and thyroid hormones.

The Error: Phenylketonuria (PKU):

Defect: A mutation in the PAH gene prevents the conversion of Phenylalanine to Tyrosine.

Consequence: Phenylalanine accumulates in the blood and brain, causing severe intellectual disability if not treated.

Traditional Treatment: Strict life-long diet avoiding protein.

2026 Therapeutic Breakthrough: As of December 2025, Otsuka and Jnana Therapeutics initiated a Global Phase 3 Clinical Trial for "Repinatrabit" (JNT-517). Unlike previous treatments that tried to fix the enzyme, this is a "transport inhibitor." It blocks the SLC6A19 transporter in the kidney, forcing the body to excrete excess Phenylalanine in urine. It is a potential game-changer, allowing patients to eat near-normal diets.

B. Branched-Chain Amino Acids (Leucine, Isoleucine, Valine)

Normal Pathway: These are metabolized in muscle (not liver) for energy. The first step involves the Branched-Chain Alpha-Ketoacid Dehydrogenase (BCKDC) complex.

The Error: Maple Syrup Urine Disease (MSUD):

Defect: Deficiency in the BCKDC complex.

Consequence: Accumulation of BCAAs and their toxic keto-acids. The urine smells like burnt sugar or maple syrup due to sotolone. It causes severe neurological damage and coma.

2026 Therapeutic Landscape: Clinical trials in late 2025 have been investigating Sodium Phenylbutyrate (traditionally used for urea cycle disorders) for MSUD. The hypothesis is that it helps lower BCAA levels by an alternate pathway, offering a buffer against the metabolic crises that threaten these patients' lives.

C. The Methionine Cycle & Homocystinuria

Normal Pathway: Methionine is converted to Cysteine. An intermediate in this pathway is Homocysteine.

The Error: Homocystinuria:

Defect: Usually a deficiency in Cystathionine beta-synthase (CBS).

Consequence: High levels of Homocysteine, which is toxic to blood vessels (causing clots/strokes) and connective tissue (causing lens dislocation in the eye and skeletal deformities similar to Marfan syndrome).

NUTRITION

Module Introduction: The New Nutritional Ecology

Welcome to the 2026 advanced module on Nutritional Biochemistry. If you think nutrition is just about counting calories or balancing macros, you are operating on outdated software. In 2026, we view nutrition through the lens of "Nutritional Ecology" and "Precision Biochemistry." It is no longer merely about fuel; it is about information. Every molecule you ingest acts as a signaling agent that talks to your DNA, modulates your gut microbiome, and dictates the structural integrity of your cell membranes.

We are moving away from the "one-size-fits-all" approach. With the rise of GLP-1 agonists reshaping how society views satiety and the 2025 ICD-11 updates redefining malnutrition, this course will take you through the biomedical engines of life, the clinical consequences of fuel failure, and the controversial metrics we use to measure it all.

1. Biomedical Importance of Nutrition

Biomedically, nutrition is the supply chain of life. Without it, the biochemical factory of the human body shuts down. But let's drill deeper than the basics. In 2026, we understand the biomedical importance of nutrition through three primary pillars: Energetics, structural integrity, and nutrigenomic signaling.

The Metabolic Currency: ATP and Coenzymes

At its core, nutrition provides the substrates—carbohydrates, lipids, and proteins—that our mitochondria burn to mint ATP (Adenosine Triphosphate). Think of ATP as the universal currency of your body. You can't pay your heart to beat or your neurons to fire without it.

The Coenzyme Connection: This is where micronutrients (vitamins and minerals) shine. They are the "workers" on the factory line. For instance, Magnesium (Mg^{2+}) is required for the stability of ATP. Without Vitamin B3 (Niacin), your body cannot form NAD^+, a critical electron carrier in the respiratory chain. You could eat all the glucose in the world, but without these micronutrient keys, the engine won't start.

Nutrigenomics: Food as Code

The most exciting development in 2026 biochemistry is Nutrigenomics. We now know that nutrients are transcription factors.

Example: Omega-3 fatty acids don't just sit in cell membranes; they enter the cell nucleus and bind to PPARs (Peroxisome Proliferator-Activated Receptors), literally turning on genes that burn fat and turning off genes that cause inflammation. When you eat, you are programming your genome.

The Microbiome Interface

We cannot talk about biomedical importance without mentioning the "second brain"—the gut microbiome. Fiber is no longer seen as just "roughage" for digestion. In 2026, we practice "Fibermaxxing" because fiber is the primary fuel for colonic bacteria, which convert it into Short-Chain Fatty Acids (SCFAs) like butyrate. Butyrate feeds the colonocytes and signals the blood-brain barrier to reduce neuroinflammation.

Biochemical Takeaway: Nutrition is the provision of molecular tools. Deficiencies are not just "low fuel"; they are missing parts in a complex machine, leading to stalled reactions and accumulation of toxic intermediates.

2. The Importance of a Balanced Diet

In the past, a "balanced diet" meant a colorful pyramid. Today, it means a Functional Matrix. The 2025/2026 nutritional landscape has shifted focus toward nutrient density and the food matrix—how nutrients are structurally bound together in whole foods versus isolated in supplements.

The Synergy of the Matrix

A balanced diet provides "Synergistic Nutrition."

Absorption Logic: Iron from spinach is poorly absorbed unless paired with Vitamin C (citrus). Fat-soluble vitamins (A, D, E, K) are useless without dietary lipids to ferry them across the intestinal wall. A balanced diet ensures these pairings happen naturally.

The GLP-1 Era: With the massive popularity of weight-management medications in 2025, the definition of a balanced diet has evolved to prioritize protein and fiber. Why? Because when appetite is suppressed, every bite must count. We are seeing a shift toward "high-efficiency" eating—smaller portions packed with essential amino acids and micronutrients to prevent muscle loss (sarcopenia).

Prevention of Chronic Disease

A balanced diet is the most powerful prophylactic drug we have.

Metabolic Flexibility: A diet balanced in complex carbohydrates and healthy fats allows the body to switch easily between burning glucose and burning fat. This flexibility is the hallmark of metabolic health and prevents Insulin Resistance (Type 2 Diabetes).

Mental Health: Emerging research links the "Western Diet" (high processed sugar/fats) to depression via neuro-inflammation. A balanced diet rich in polyphenols (from berries, tea, dark chocolate) acts as an antioxidant shield for the brain.

3. Clinical Abnormalities Associated with Nutritional Imbalance

When the biochemical supply chain breaks, clinical pathology ensues. The 2025 ICD-11 updates have refined how we classify these disorders, moving beyond simple weight measures to look at function.
Undernutrition: The Starvation States

Despite global obesity, undernutrition remains a critical issue. We divide this into two classic biochemical failures:

Marasmus (Energy Failure): This is total calorie deprivation. The body shifts into "autocannibalism," stripping down skeletal muscle to free up amino acids for gluconeogenesis (making sugar for the brain). The patient appears "wasted" (skin and bones) but alert.

Kwashiorkor (Protein Failure): This is insidious. The patient might have enough calories (from starchy fillers) but lacks protein. Without amino acids, the liver cannot synthesize Albumin, the protein that keeps fluid in the blood vessels.

The Result: Fluid leaks out into the tissues, causing edema (swelling) and a distended belly (ascites). The immune system collapses because antibodies are made of protein.

Overnutrition: The Toxicity of Excess

Overnutrition is not just "being fat"; it is a state of chronic cellular stress.

Metabolic Syndrome: A cluster of conditions—high blood pressure, high blood sugar, excess body fat around the waist, and abnormal cholesterol levels. Biochemically, the adipocytes (fat cells) become "sick" and start releasing inflammatory cytokines (IL-6, TNF-alpha) instead of regulating energy. This leads to systemic inflammation.

Micronutrient Toxicity: You can have too much of a good thing. For example, Hypervitaminosis A can cause liver damage and intracranial pressure. This is becoming more common with the rise of aggressive supplementation.

Specific Deficiency Disorders

Scurvy (Vitamin C deficiency): Without Vitamin C, the enzyme prolyl hydroxylase fails. Collagen cannot cross-link. The result? Bleeding gums, loose teeth, and wounds that won't heal.

Beriberi (Thiamine/B1 deficiency): Common in alcoholics or high-refined-rice diets. Without B1, the body cannot convert pyruvate to acetyl-CoA. The neurological system crashes (confusion, ataxia).

4. The Importance of Body Mass Index (BMI)

Here is where we need to be critical. Body Mass Index (BMI) has been the "gold standard" for decades, but in 2026, it is viewed as a "blunt instrument."

What is it?

BMI is a simple heuristic: a calculation of weight in relation to height.

BMI=height(m)2weight(kg)
Why is it still important?

Despite its flaws, BMI is important for population-level screening. It is cheap, non-invasive, and universally understood. In large datasets, high BMI correlates strongly with risks of cardiovascular disease, diabetes, and certain cancers. It is a "red flag" that prompts further investigation.

The 2026 Critique: The "BMI-Plus" Era

In 2026, we acknowledge that BMI lies. It cannot distinguish between:

Lean Mass vs. Fat Mass: A bodybuilder with 8% body fat might have a BMI of 32 (Obese) because muscle is denser than fat.

Visceral vs. Subcutaneous Fat: It doesn't tell us where the fat is. "Skinny fat" individuals (normal BMI but high visceral fat wrapped around organs) are at higher metabolic risk than "fit fat" individuals (high BMI but high muscle mass and subcutaneous fat).

Current Clinical Standard: We now use BMI-Plus. We combine BMI with Waist Circumference and Bioelectrical

Impedance to get a true picture of health. If BMI is the "check engine" light, these other metrics are the mechanic's diagnostic tool.

5. Calculating BMI: A Practical Guide

Let's get into the math. The formula is universal for adults, regardless of gender, though the interpretation of the health risk might vary slightly based on body composition (women naturally carry more essential fat).

Formula:
BMI=(Height in Meters)2Weight in Kilograms
Case Study A: The "Average" Male

Subject: Mark, 35 years old.

Weight: 85 kg

Height: 1.8 meters (approx 5'11")

Calculation:

Square the height: $1.8 \times 1.8 = 3.24$

Divide weight by squared height: $85/3.24 = 26.23$

Result: Mark has a BMI of 26.2. Classification: Overweight (Range is 25.0 – 29.9).

2026 Analysis: We would ask Mark for his waist measurement. If it's under 40 inches, he might just be muscular. If it's over, the BMI is accurate regarding risk.

Case Study B: The "Petite" Female

Subject: Sarah, 28 years old.

Weight: 50 kg

Height: 1.6 meters (approx 5'3")

Calculation:

Square the height: $1.6 \times 1.6 = 2.56$

Divide weight by squared height: $50/2.56 = 19.53$

Result: Sarah has a BMI of 19.5. Classification: Normal Weight (Range is 18.5 – 24.9).

2026 Analysis: While "normal," we ensure she isn't sarcopenic (low muscle mass), which is a risk even at healthy weights.

Case Study C: The "Obese" Classification

Subject: John, 45 years old.

Weight: 110 kg

Height: 1.75 meters

Calculation:

Square the height: $1.75 \times 1.75 = 3.0625$

Divide weight by squared height: $110/3.0625 = 35.9$

Result: John has a BMI of 35.9. Classification: Obesity Class II (Range is 35.0 – 39.9).

ENDOCRINOLOGY

1. Introduction to Endocrinology

Endocrinology is not merely the study of glands; it is the study of communication. If the nervous system is the body's hard-wired biological internet, the endocrine system is its Wi-Fi—a wireless, chemical signaling network that permeates every tissue to maintain homeostasis.

Defining Hormones Biochemically, a hormone is a chemical messenger synthesized by specialized cells, secreted directly into the bloodstream (or interstitial fluid), and transported to distant target organs where it elicits a specific biological response at very low concentrations (10−9 to 10−12 M).

In the context of 2026 biochemistry, our definition has expanded. We no longer view hormones simply as "glandular secretions." We now understand them as "information molecules." Any molecule—whether a peptide from the gut, a steroid from the adrenal cortex, or a cytokine from adipose tissue—that the organism uses to convey metabolic status to other tissues qualifies as a hormone.

2. Classification of Hormones

To understand how hormones work, we must first classify them by their chemical nature. This is not just a filing system; the chemistry of a hormone dictates how it travels in blood, where its receptor is located, and how long it lasts.

Group I: Lipophilic Hormones (The Nuclear Travelers)

Chemistry: Derived from cholesterol (steroids) or tyrosine (thyroid hormones).

Solubility: Low solubility in water; they require transport proteins (e.g., Cortisol Binding Globulin, Thyroxine Binding Globulin) to swim through the bloodstream.

Half-life: Long (hours to days).

Examples: Cortisol, Aldosterone, Testosterone, Estrogen, T3, T4.

Key Feature: They can cross the cell membrane freely.

Group II: Hydrophilic Hormones (The Membrane Knockers)

Chemistry: Amino acid derivatives, peptides, and large proteins.

Solubility: Highly soluble in plasma; they travel unbound.

Half-life: Short (minutes).

Examples: Insulin, Glucagon, Epinephrine, Growth Hormone, ACTH.

Key Feature: They cannot cross the lipid bilayer of the cell; they must knock on the door (bind to surface receptors).

3. General Characteristics & Mechanism of Action

In 2026, we categorize hormonal action into two distinct pathways: the Genomic (slow, sustained) and the Non-Genomic (rapid, transient).

A. Mechanism of Lipophilic Hormones (Genomic Action)

These hormones act as "molecular keys" that unlock genetic potential.

Entry: The hormone diffuses across the plasma membrane.

Binding: It binds to a specific intracellular receptor (cytosolic or nuclear).

Transformation: The Hormone-Receptor (H-R) complex undergoes a conformational change (dimerization).

DNA Interaction: The complex enters the nucleus and binds to specific DNA sequences called Hormone Response Elements (HREs) using "Zinc Finger" motifs.

Transcription: This binding recruits co-activators (like SRC-1) or co-repressors, altering the transcription of mRNA.

Result: New proteins are synthesized.

2026 Update: Recent research highlights Non-Genomic Actions of steroid and thyroid hormones. For example, Thyroid Hormone (T3) has been found to bind to integrin receptors ($\alpha v\beta 3$) on the cell surface to trigger rapid vasodilation via the MAPK pathway, bypassing the nucleus entirely.

B. Mechanism of Hydrophilic Hormones (Signal Transduction)

Since these cannot enter the cell, they use a "second messenger" system—a molecular relay race.

1. The G-Protein Coupled Receptor (GPCR) System:

The First Messenger: The hormone (e.g., Epinephrine) binds to the surface receptor.

The Transducer: This activates a G-protein (specifically the Gs subunit).

The Effector: Gs stimulates the enzyme Adenylate Cyclase.

The Second Messenger: Adenylate Cyclase converts ATP into cyclic AMP (cAMP).

The Cascade: cAMP activates Protein Kinase A (PKA), which phosphorylates downstream enzymes, turning them on or off.

2. The Receptor Tyrosine Kinase (RTK) System (e.g., Insulin):

The receptor itself is an enzyme. When insulin binds, the receptor autophosphorylates (adds phosphate groups to itself).

This creates a docking site for proteins like IRS-1 (Insulin Receptor Substrate), triggering a cascade (PI3K/Akt pathway) that moves glucose transporters to the surface.

4. Detailed Metabolic Roles of Specific Glands
A. The Hypothalamus: The CEO of Metabolism

The hypothalamus is the command center where the nervous system meets the endocrine system. It doesn't just "release hormones"; it integrates environmental data (light, stress, temperature) with metabolic data (glucose, leptin levels).

Chemistry: It produces small peptides known as "Releasing Hormones" (e.g., TRH, CRH, GnRH).

Mechanism: These peptides travel down the hypophyseal portal system (a private blood vessel highway) directly to the anterior pituitary. They act via GPCRs ($Ca2+$/IP3 pathway) to stimulate secretion.

2026 Insight: We now understand the Epigenetic Plasticity of the hypothalamus. Environmental factors like high-sugar diets can methylate the DNA of hypothalamic neurons (specifically POMC and AgRP neurons), permanently altering their sensitivity to satiety signals. This "metabolic imprinting" is a key focus of modern obesity treatment.

B. The Pituitary Gland: The Master Conductor

The pituitary translates the hypothalamus's whispered commands into loud, systemic signals.

Anterior Pituitary:

Growth Hormone (GH): A protein hormone that works via the JAK/STAT pathway. It stimulates the liver to produce IGF-1.

Metabolic Role: It is "diabetogenic"—it saves glucose for the brain by forcing muscle/fat to burn fatty acids (lipolysis) and inhibiting glucose uptake.

ACTH: Derived from a massive precursor protein called POMC (Pro-opiomelanocortin). It stimulates the adrenal cortex.

Posterior Pituitary:

Stores Oxytocin and Vasopressin (ADH). ADH regulates water retention by inserting aquaporin channels in the kidney.

C. The Thyroid Gland: The Metabolic Throttle

Located in the neck, the thyroid dictates the Basal Metabolic Rate (BMR).

Chemistry: T4 (Thyroxine) and T3 (Triiodothyronine) are iodinated tyrosine derivatives.

Biosynthesis: Requires the protein Thyroglobulin and the enzyme Thyroid Peroxidase (TPO), which iodinates tyrosine residues.

Mechanism: T4 is the "pro-hormone" (storage form). Once it enters a cell, enzymes called Deiodinases strip an iodine to convert it into T3, the active form. T3 enters the nucleus to upregulate genes for metabolic machinery.

Metabolic Role:

Carbohydrates: Increases glucose absorption from the gut.

Lipids: Stimulates the breakdown of cholesterol (increases LDL receptors).

Energy: Increases the number and activity of Mitochondria and stimulates the Na^+/K^+-ATPase pump, consuming ATP to generate heat (thermogenesis).

D. The Adrenal Gland: Stress and Survival

The adrenal gland is two glands in one: the outer Cortex and the inner Medulla.

1. Adrenal Cortex (Steroids):

Glucocorticoids (Cortisol):

Mechanism: Genomic action via the Glucocorticoid Receptor (GR).

Metabolic Role: Cortisol is the "famine hormone." It assumes you are starving or injured.

Gluconeogenesis: It breaks down muscle protein into amino acids to make new glucose in the liver.

Lipolysis: It mobilizes fatty acids.

Anti-inflammatory: It inhibits NF-κB, a master switch for inflammation.

Mineralocorticoids (Aldosterone): Regulates blood pressure by retaining Sodium (Na^+) and dumping Potassium (K^+) in the kidneys.

2. Adrenal Medulla (Catecholamines):

Epinephrine (Adrenaline):

Chemistry: Synthesized from Tyrosine.

Mechanism: Acts via GPCRs (α and β adrenergic receptors).

Metabolic Role: The "Fight or Flight" response. It triggers immediate glycogen breakdown (glycogenolysis) in the liver and muscle to flood the blood with fuel.

E. The Pancreas: The Fuel Gauge

The Islets of Langerhans within the pancreas act as the body's primary energy sensor, maintaining glucose between 70-100 mg/dL.

Insulin (The Storage Hormone):

Chemistry: A peptide of 51 amino acids (A-chain and B-chain linked by disulfide bridges). Secreted as a hexamer (6 units) but active as a monomer.

Mechanism: Binds the Insulin Receptor (RTK). The 2026 understanding emphasizes the structural shift of the receptor from an "inverted-V" to a "T-shape" upon binding, which brings the internal kinase domains together for activation.

Metabolic Role:

Carbs: Translocates GLUT4 transporters to the cell surface of muscle/fat to act as doors for glucose entry.

Lipids: Activates Lipoprotein Lipase (LPL) to store fat; inhibits hormone-sensitive lipase (stops fat breakdown).

Protein: Stimulates amino acid uptake (anabolic).

Glucagon (The Retrieval Hormone):

Acts largely on the liver via cAMP to reverse insulin's effects: stimulates glycogenolysis and gluconeogenesis during fasting.

5. Conclusion & Future Outlook

To summarize, the endocrine system is a highly sophisticated masterpiece of biochemical engineering. From the pulsatile secretions of the hypothalamus to the genomic transcription initiated by thyroid hormones, every step is regulated by exquisite feedback loops.

As we look at the landscape of biochemistry in 2026, the boundary between "hormone" and "drug" is blurring. We are seeing the rise of Dual-Agonists (like Tirzepatide variants) that hit both GLP-1 and GIP receptors to treat obesity with unprecedented efficacy. We are mapping the Epigenetic changes in the hypothalamus that dictate metabolic set-points.

The future of endocrinology lies not just in replacing missing hormones, but in fine-tuning the sensitivity of their receptors and understanding the "crosstalk" between organs—how the bone talks to the pancreas (via osteocalcin) and how the gut talks to the brain.

About Author

Azhar ul Haque Sario is a bestselling author and data scientist with a remarkable record of achievement. This Cambridge alumnus brings a wealth of knowledge to his work, holding an MBA (SZABIST), ACCA (Knowledge Level - FTMS College Malaysia and London College of Accountancy, London), BBA, and several Google certifications, including specializations in Google Data Analytics, Google Digital Marketing & E-commerce, and Google Project Management.

With ten years of business experience, Azhar combines practical expertise with his impressive academic background to craft insightful books. His prolific writing has resulted in an astounding 2810 published titles, earning him the record for the maximum Kindle editions and paperback books published by an individual author in one year, awarded by Asia Books of Records in 2024.

ORCID: https://orcid.org/0009-0004-8629-830X
Azhar.sario@hotmail.co.uk
https://www.linkedin.com/in/azharulhaquesario/

www.ingramcontent.com/pod-product-compliance
Lightning Source LLC
Chambersburg PA
CBHW031347230926
51848CB00002B/416
9783384797179